The Roots
of Healing

The Roots
of Healing

A Woman's Book of Herbs

by Deb Soule

Illustrated by Susan Szwed

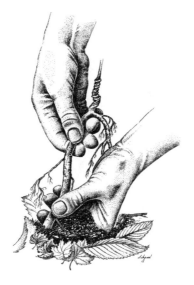

A CITADEL PRESS BOOK
Published by Carol Publishing Group

Carol Publishing Group Edition, 1996

A Citadel Press Book
Published by Carol Publishing Group
Citadel Press is a registered trademark of Carol Communications, Inc.

Editorial, sales and distribution, rights and permissions inquiries should be addressed Carol Publishing Group, 120 Enterprise Avenue, Secaucus, N.J. 07094

In Canada: Canadian Manda Group, One Atlantic Avenue, Suite 105, Toronto, Ontario M6K 3E7

Carol Publishing Group books may be purchased in bulk at special discounts for sales promotions, fund-raising, or educational purposes. Special editions can be created to specifications. For details, contact Special Sales Department, 120 Enterprise Avenue, Secaucus, N.J. 07094

Manufactured in the United States of America
10 9 8 7 6 5 4 3 2

Library of Congress Cataloging-in-Publication Data

Soule, Deb.
    The roots of healing : a woman's book of herbs / by Deb Soule;
Illustrated by Susan Szwed.
        p.   cm.
"A Citadel Press book."
ISBN 0-8065-1578-3
1. Generative organs, Female–Diseases–Treatment. 2. Herbs–
Therapeutic use. 3. Self medication. 4. Gynecology–Popular
works. I. Title.
RG129.H47S66   1994
615'.321'082—dc20   94-20350
                                                      CIP

Dedication

This book is dedicated to the following Elder women who significantly touched my life: Adele Dawson, Marija Gimbutas, Helen Nearing, and Katherine Soule Foster. I stand taller and stronger today because of their influence and firm support.

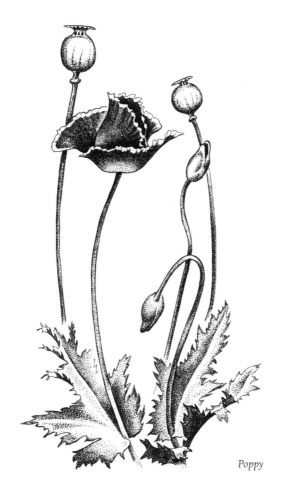

Poppy

Contents

Acknowledgments

I am deeply grateful to the many people who have helped me birth this book. First, I acknowledge the women herbalists who courageously walked this path before me. Their rich stories and wisdom, most of which was passed on orally or left in gardens, is being woven back together by contemporary women.

I bow to my grandmother, Katherine Soule Foster, who taught me how to carefully see and hear with more than my eyes and ears, and reopened the magic of the natural world to me when I was five years old. Katherine's respect and love for plants, birds, and animals is the foundation in which my understanding of healing is firmly rooted.

I am grateful to the dozens of women who, over several years, have shared their health problems and herbal success stories with me. These experiences validate the effectiveness of herbs and allow the wisdom to be passed on. Special thanks to the medicine plants themselves, who continue to bless us with their gifts that heal body and spirit.

To the following teachers I have been graced with in my life I give thanks: Adele Dawson, Helen Nearing, Mary Bove, Doug Elliot, Sara Smith, Ed Smith, Amanda McQuade Crawford, Rosemary Gladstar, Juliette de Bairacli Levy, Cascade Anderson Geller, AmyLee, and Norma Myers. Special thanks to Thich Nhat Hanh, Vietnamese Buddhist Zen teacher, for the practice of the precepts and mindfulness teachings that guide my work; to my friends in Nepal for introducing me to Green Tara; to Her Eminence Jetsun Kushok for the Green Tara initiation; and to Marija Gimbutas for helping reawaken my knowing of the Goddess.

Many thanks to Selkie O'Mira, Helen Caddie-Larcenia, Rose Crandall, and Sheila Garrett, who cared for the lab at Avena Botanicals during the initial stages of this book, and for the Avena "fairies," Kimber Lee Clark, Gwen, Delia Mae Farris, Cathy Webb, Susy Ellis, and Carol Begin, whose support and love helped me through the final stages of writing. Special thanks to Betsy Hart, M.D., who offered me tremendous emotional support and assistance in the lab at Avena and also carefully read the manuscript for medical correctness.

Many thanks to Anne Dellenbaugh; Suzanne Richman; Patricia Reis; Hart Brent; Matty Becker; Susan Thomas; Sue Farrell; Kate Norris; Mary Lynn Garner, N.D.; Devra Krassner, N.D.; Susan Lie-Nielson; Maggie Davis; Peaches Bass; Ruth Lockart; Priscilla Skerry, N.D.; Tori Hudson, N.D.; Christine Northrup, M.D.; Arifa Boehler; Shep Erhart from Maine Coast Sea Vegetables; Dee Webster; Kathaeryn Walker; C. R. Lawn; David Winston; David Hart; Chris Bey; Beth Edmonds; Cynthia Phinney; Susan Plourde, Pat and Lester Soule, Patrick Giantonio, Nancy Hanrahan; Earth John; and Judy and Linsey Powers for help and support with various aspects of the manuscript.

I am grateful to Elizabeth Garber-Baldwin, my acupuncturist, for her wise and tender touch; to the women in my full-moon group, who witnessed this book's unfolding over many moons; to Rebecca Willow, Sharon Hayes-Whitney, Jean Wakem, and Carmen Brochu for helping me care for Avena's gardens; and to the Earth Sisters who dare to keep this herbal tradition alive.

Special thanks to my agent, Cheryl Seal, who believed in me and this book; to Sue Szwed for her beautiful illustrations; and to my editor, Denise O'Sullivan. And thanks to my friends Deborah Wiggs, Selkie O'Mira, Eremi and Karinate Amabebe, Helen Caddie-Larcenia, and Mochi, my dog, for letting themselves become illustrations for this book.

Mochi was my closest companion and hour-by-hour support team throughout the writing process. She lay near me as I typed and every few hours encouraged me to roll around on the floor or go outside with her, always a benefit to my brain and spirit. My cat, Osha, often sat in my lap and kept me company as I typed. Her wild spirit and soft paws kept me from disappearing into the computer. Though she disappeared before this book came to completion, her feline wisdom is woven between the lines and lives on in my heart.

I thank Alexandra Merrill for her support and understanding of women's group process, which inspired, challenged, and fed me throughout the writing of this book. I often found myself erasing a word or phrase, looking for new ways to express my woman heart. I apologize for any words or statements that may seem inappropriate or outdated. Unlearning old ways of communicating is an ongoing process. The written word is never final. The information and ideas in this book will continue to change, just as plants and women do.

Last, I give my love and appreciation to my partner, Abby Morrison, whose constant love, support, and belief in me are a blessing in my life. She continues to be the tree in our household, firmly rooted and willing to bend with the breezes.

To the Reader: The author is donating a percentage of her royalties to help set up a teaching clinic in Maine that will offer free herbal and homeopathic care to low-income women and families. Another percentage is being donated to help set up a wildlife rehabilitation center in Maine that will use herbs and homeopathy.

Herbs have a long history of being used for medicinal purposes around the world. The information about the herbs listed in this book comes from many herbalists' observations and years of practice. The suggestions and procedures in this book are meant to supplement your overall health. It is important to seek out appropriate medical care when needed.

The author and publishers are not responsible for the use or misuse of the information presented in this book.

The Roots
of Healing

Introduction

A garden, small or large, like a nuclear or extended family, gives us a protected, friendly place to grow–not only to grow herbs in a way compatible with nature, but to grow in our own psychic awareness, to cultivate our potential for being sensitive and responsible citizens of the planet and grateful caretakers of our inherited treasures.[1]

–ADELE DAWSON

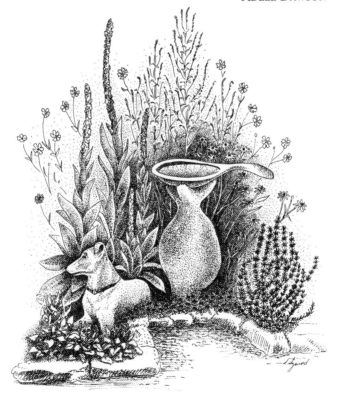

When I was a young child growing up in rural Maine, my grandmother introduced me to the beauty and magic of plants and animals. I spent hours wandering through nearby fields, woods, and abandoned apple orchards, delighting in the wildflowers, birch trees, ferns, and fragrant apple blossoms.

At the age of fifteen I began gardening. Shortly afterward I learned that many of the wild and cultivated plants I cherished could be used for healing. Some place deep inside me remembered this. I began to seek out people who knew about herbs and to read any herb book I could find. For nearly a decade I planted gardens and gathered the wild herbs that grew wherever I lived. In 1984 I returned to Maine to build my home and to plant the herb gardens I had dreamed of, and to create Avena Botanicals, an herbal apothecary specializing in remedies made from local wild herbs and those grown in my organic gardens.

As Avena's shelves and gardens and workshops expanded, the seeds for a woman's herb book were planted. The information in this book has been collected over the twenty years I have been growing and using herbs and working closely with both knowledgeable teachers and women in need of guidance. It is in our willingness to help each other and tell our stories that the herbal tradition has been kept alive.

I chose to write a book for women because of my love for herbs and my commitment to helping improve the quality of women's lives. This book is written from a very personal perspective, drawing on my own experiences and feminist beliefs. Most of my teachers are of European origin because my mother's roots are European. I cannot speak for the women healers and herbalists whose rich and varied traditions, remedies, and rituals are different from mine. I pass on the traditions and knowledge that have been passed on to me.

Herbal medicine is women's medicine. The village herbalist, often a woman whose knowledge came from her mother or grandmother, carefully collected the local herbs and dispensed them to those in need. The village herbalist is an important image, archetype, for women to reclaim today, whether we live in the country or city. The gentle nourishing ways of women and herbs are desperately needed in these times when hopelessness and despair are on the rise. Herbs offer us hope, beauty, and healing and give us the opportunity to create an intimate relationship with the Earth—one based on mutual respect, care, and love.

It is my belief that relearning herbal wisdom connects us to the women throughout the ages who have used plants for medicine. It does not matter whether you have ever known an herbalist; reconnecting with this timeless tradition of women herbalists can help us feel whole again. Too many of us have been uprooted from our homes, our motherlands, our blood ancestors, and their traditions. Making relationships with plants and trees reunites us with Earth and reminds us to acknowledge the women who went before us and gathered the herbs on the land we now walk upon.

Herbs are valuable allies in our quest to enrich our lives. Approach them thoughtfully, respectfully, and with a willingness to learn. There is no reason to fear them. Once you have befriended even one herb, you will be presented with an enduring relationship that will be a constant source of wisdom and joy.

Many of the herbs discussed in this book grow wild in the northeastern United States and are the same ones I grew up with. Some originally came from Europe and some are native. Others are easy to cultivate, depending on your location. Specific planting, harvesting, and processing information is included, especially for those women whose access to commercially prepared herbal remedies is limited because of financial resources or rural lifestyles and for women who love, or long, to garden. If you do not have land to garden, check with your local town or city planning board or garden club about obtaining a community garden plot. If you are unable or do not wish to grow or collect herbs, you can refer to the resource list at the end of the book for a list of sources of high quality organic and wild-harvested herbs.

What you will discover in this book are simple and practical herbal guidelines along with many words of hope and kindness

that have helped me and many other women nourish and heal ourselves and deepen our connection with the moon and Earth. Also
included are reminders of the injustices women face every day.
Because a woman's health is directly connected to her experiences,
and women everywhere are confirming the fact that poverty, sexual
abuse, racism, and other forms of oppression are adversely affecting
the quality of their health, I could not write a woman's herbal without addressing some of these conditions. They are conditions that
herbs alone cannot heal. Knowing a woman has experienced sexual abuse, or an abortion, and now has a uterine fibroid or is having
difficulty getting pregnant can be useful information when helping
her to release the trauma she has held within her body. Telling our
stories enables us to be better equipped to help ourselves and each
other.

Throughout the book I have made specific references to lesbian health issues along with including a section on lesbian health.
Lesbian and bisexual women's health issues are all too commonly
ignored or not taken seriously by the medical profession and society at large. The result is a lack of respectful and educated health
care providers for lesbians.

I have found in working with women that most of us never
learned as young girls how to nourish ourselves. It is absurd to
expect that women who grow up in a society that often devalues
and abuses women should automatically know how to love and
care for themselves. Learning how to accept and love ourselves is
an ongoing process and essential for our overall health and happiness.

Herbs alone cannot eliminate the false and hurtful beliefs
many of us have internalized. These attitudes interfere with our
abilities to love and care for ourselves and set us up for "dis-eases"
such as eating disorders, depression, alcoholism, and workaholism.
(I spell disease as *dis-ease* for health conditions that I believe are the
result of a woman receiving little or no positive affirmation while
growing up. Because of this, many women are not at ease in their
bodies and this dis-ease sometimes manifests itself as some form of
illness.) Addressing traumatic childhood experiences and the effect
society's oppressive attitudes toward women have had on us is an
important step to take in relearning self-healing. Women's support

groups, counseling, homeopathy, acupuncture, body work, meditation, dream therapy, dance therapy, journal writing, and twelve-step programs are some channels that can facilitate deep emotional shifts within us. As we heal, our minds become clearer and our hearts less fearful of living joyfully and fully.

It is my hope that as the face of medicine changes in the United States, which it must, because fewer and fewer people can meet the rising costs of conventional health care, herbal medicine will be accepted and made available to any person who wants it. Despite the orthodox medical community's reluctance to endorse herbal remedies, we herbalists continue to practice, putting our concerns for people and animals first. Some of us are bridging medical gaps by working with doctors and nurses, blending the best of herbal and allopathic medicine whenever possible.

There are specific allopathic drugs and medical techniques that, when used wisely, are beneficial. Certain antibiotics, surgical procedures, and diagnostic techniques have improved the quality of many people's lives. We must remember, however, that allopathic medicine, which is essentially the practice of curing by opposing symptoms, is, in reality, the alternative medicine, not herbal medicine. After all, the effectiveness of Western drugs has a much shorter history than that of herbal medicine. And the cruel and violent testing done on animals to prove the efficacy of allopathic drugs is a practice I and many others deplore.

There is more talk about preventive health care these days. Daily exercise, good food, meditation, rest, clean water, and time spent in nature are essential for our health. Yet we are at risk of seeing these things only as means to get healthy, instead of being things that offer us pleasure and peace of mind. All of the above things can and do nourish the body when embraced in a balanced and not overly fanatical way.

I am also sensitive to the fact that the inequitable and unjust economic situation in the United States enables people with money to take better care of themselves (even though many do not). The cost of organic food, good quality vitamins and mineral supplements, and appointments with conventional and holistic health practitioners is prohibitive to many people. I dream of community-supported organic farms and holistic health centers rising up everywhere so that the general population has access to good quality food, herbs, and health care.

WELCOME TO THE WORLD OF HERBS

Plants are made up of a myriad of chemical constituents, including alkaloids, sugars, carbohydrates, resins, essential oils, and glycosides. A plant in its whole form has a very different response in the body than it does when it is taken apart and/or chemically synthesized into a drug. Herbs grown, gathered, and prepared respectfully embody the plant's life energy, which I believe is essential for healing to occur.

A fun and effective way to learn to identify herbs is by spending time with an herbalist, a local plant enthusiast, or a botanist. The more you are among plants, the more familiar they will become to you and the easier they will be to identify. Learn the plants that grow in your dooryard. Knowing ten local herbs well will enable you to fill your home medicine chest. If you are interested in recognizing a large number of plants, prepare yourself for a lifelong adventure.

It is imperative when collecting herbs for edible and medicinal purposes that you harvest the correct plant. Make sure you know the Latin name of any plant you intend to pick in the wild or cultivate in your garden. Some common names of plants can vary greatly or overlap with others, depending on your region, the guide you are using, or the botanist you consult. Check Latin names even when you buy seeds or plants. For example, calendula is often referred to colloquially as "pot marigold," yet is not actually a marigold at all. *Calendula officinalis* is the genus (*Calendula*) and species (*officinalis*) that you want for medicinal purposes. Hybrid varieties of calendula and other herbs are sold commercially and you want to avoid them. Most herb books, seed catalogs, and nurseries list Latin names. All the herbs in this book are listed alphabetically with both common and Latin names in the appendix.

Understanding and using herbs is both an art and a science. Begin using herbs for minor problems. This will build your trust in their effectiveness. Select herbs that address the needs of the whole person, not just the symptoms of the dis-ease. Western medical technology has moved our society farther and farther away from believing in nature's ability to heal. Using herbs can help us to weave nature's timeless wisdom back into our daily lives and to restore the balance and harmony that has been lost.

The many phases and transitions in our lives are the rich material that opens us to more fully understanding who we are as women living on this Earth. The chapters in this book follow a woman's spiritual journey; how we learn to nourish ourselves; our ability to digest food and events in our life; our relationship with the many aspects of being a woman such as menstruation, menopause, growing older; and the wisdom that comes with reconnecting with the moon and Earth. We heal as we connect with our inner selves, with our ancestral roots, with our communities; as we find our voices, reclaim our bodies, and rejoice in being alive. Herbs are friends to have along on your journey. They embody Earth's wisdom, vitality, and beauty and reflect back to us our own beauty and goodness.

May this book be a friend to you, one whose words can in some way help soften old wounds, whose pages are like a soft bed of chamomile flowers to rest upon, and whose essence helps you remember the wisdom you carry within. May your journey with herbs bring you endless joy and delight and may you in turn keep passing their teachings on.

Deb Soule
May 1994
Rockland, Maine

1

Remembering Our Roots

For each of us as women, there is a dark place within where, hidden and growing, our true spirit rises. . . . These places of possibility within ourselves are dark because they are ancient and hidden; they have survived and grown strong through that darkness. Within these deep places, each one of us holds an incredible reserve of creativity and power, of unexamined and unrecorded emotion and feeling. The woman's place of power within each of us is neither white nor surface; it is dark, it is ancient, and it is deep.

—AUDRE LORDE

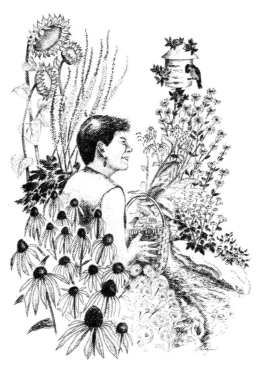

Women have long been the keepers of herbal knowledge and other wise medicine ways. There have always been, and are still those among us who know how to identify, gather, and use herbs for medicine. We understand that the primary life force of Earth is contained within the plants. We trust in Earth's healing abilities and therefore have continued to call upon herbs for nutritional, medicinal, and spiritual help.

We are the healers who prepare teas, baths, and poultices; set bones; and stitch wounds. We attend births and administer both fertility-promoting and contraceptive herbs. We listen to people's troubles and give counsel to those who ask for help. We also acknowledge that death is a part of life's journey and are present to assist others as they pass from this world. We offer songs and prayers in our work, healing from our hearts with deep respect and compassion for all living beings.

We are known in our communities as herbalists, midwives, witches, nurses, teachers, doctors, hospice workers, curanderas, and wise women. Our healing skills are noninvasive, for we know the body heals itself when given proper nourishment and support. Our reverence for the mysteries of birth, life, death, and renewal guides us to live in harmony with nature, closely following her rhythms. We are connected to the changing seasons, the weather, and the cycles of the moon. We are not afraid to enter the unknown and dark places within ourselves, for we know seeds of wisdom sprout there.

We have continued to practice our healing arts despite centuries of persecution by religious organizations, governments, and medical establishments. Long ago, the wise women who survived went underground in order to keep the traditions alive. Today, the whisperings of ancient women are being heard by many women around the world. Deep inside we remember that all life, including our own, is sacred. We are once again gathering together to offer support and information and to challenge the dysfunctions and violence in homes and communities. We are redefining ourselves as powerful, gifted, and intelligent. We are recreating rituals, songs, and dances that honor Earth and women. We are reclaiming our rights to care for ourselves and others. We never completely lost the crafts we practiced and the gentle wisdom we offered others. We have carried women's wisdom in our cellular memories, in the fabric of our beings, in our wombs, generation after generation. Our bodies are vessels that preserved the knowledge when it was not safe to speak. We have always been the healers. And this is still true.

The remembering journey often begins when we find ourselves asking, Who am I? and What does it mean to be a woman living in the twentieth century? The process of rediscovery occurs as we peel away the layers and lies that have kept us from honoring and connecting with the daughter, mother, and crone (a woman who knows and trusts her inner strength, wisdom, and power) aspects within ourselves. In this process we mend the wounds that have alienated us from ourselves as women. This journey can be painful, filled with feelings of shame, abandonment, fear, anger, rage, deep sadness, and grief. As we move through the layers, our relationship to painful emotions and experiences changes: We no longer allow them to control us.

THE ROOTS OF HEALING

Learning to nurture ourselves often begins when we let ourselves feel unconditionally loved. I began to feel this sense of love as I immersed myself into the world of herbs. Over time I realized that a presence of unconditional love was emanating from Earth herself through the herbs. This presence, I came to realize, is divine female wisdom, the Great Goddess. Patricia Reis writes in *Through the Goddess: A Woman's Way of Healing*

> An awareness of the Goddess helps to awaken women to ways in which our deepest female body experiences, our psyche's realities, and our spiritual quests are all related. It is critically important, I believe, to bring an awareness of the Goddess forward now, because she adds a needed dimension of dignity and meaning to women's current struggle for self-becoming.[1]

"Venus of Laussel," (25,000–20,000 B.C.E.) carved in limestone over the entrance to a cave in Laussel, Dordogne, France. Her left hand touches her belly and her right hand holds a horned crescent marked with thirteen incisions, representing the number of moon cycles in a solar year.

A feeling that something long lost in me had been found came to me as I began to see images of breasts, hips, vaginas, and full pregnant bellies in the swelling blossoms, the burls on trees, the trumpets of flowers, and the soft mounds of moss. I found myself planting gardens with these shapes before I fully understood the underlying meaning of these images so deeply encoded in my psyche. Now I know that my passion for gardening, working with seeds, moist soil, and living plants, has helped me reclaim my woman's body and has guided me as I have made my way back to myself and to Earth.

One night, some time after I had begun writing this book, I had a vivid dream that woke me up. In this dream I saw myself sitting cross-legged on soft, rich soil with two women whom I have met, one whose lineage is Micmac (a Native American tribe whose homeland is the areas now referred to as northern Maine, New Brunswick, and Nova Scotia) and the other whose lineage is Portuguese, French, and English. Together, we were weaving a beautiful, womb-shaped basket. I sensed this image was very important to what I was trying to do in writing my book. I realized that the womb-shaped basket symbolized my belief that all women are sacred vessels with rich traditions and unique abilities to create beauty, and that there can be powerful unity in our diversity. Together we can mold strong vessels filled with women's wisdom that cannot be destroyed by fear, hatred, ignorance, or distrust. Our vessels can cross the racial, ethnic, and class boundaries that have kept us separated from each other. We are all of this Earth. And we share being women as the common vessel.

The thoughtful words and actions and creative work of women are deeply needed in these times of suffering. One in eight women in the United States is challenged with breast cancer. Indigenous peoples and the natural world are rapidly being destroyed by clear-cutting, pesticides, toxic dumps, and farming practices that deplete the soil and pollute the water. Our willingness to continuously reevaluate our own lifestyles and prejudices and join with others to find creative, sustainable, and compassionate solutions is necessary for the survival of all life. This is a time that calls for a peaceful yet powerful commitment to healing.

Herbs are gifts that teach and heal. Through them we can learn to hear the whisperings of Earth herself. Sit quietly with them in the wild or in a garden. Listen for their songs. Watch them grow and change throughout the seasons. Feel, smell, and touch them gently. Lie with your belly to the earth and observe the herbs at their own level instead of always hovering above them. Move a little slower. Bathe in the full-moon light a little more often. Laugh a little louder. Let yourself remember the wise woman who lives within you.

A Brief History of the European Wise Women from the Witch Burnings to the Present

Somewhere deep in women's psyches—in our cells, in our bones— we remember the witch burnings, which began around the twelfth century in Europe. Knowledge of this history helps women be wiser today about who we allow to be our health care providers and what healing methods we choose. The effects of the witch-burning times are still with us today as women continue to struggle to have economic, spiritual, emotional, and medical freedoms.

The final years of the Middle Ages were a time of incredible strife, sickness, war, and ecological destruction throughout Europe. Overcrowded villages and cities, severe crop failures, and generally unsanitary conditions led to increases in disease and death. The plague, also known as the Black Death, raged across Europe.

Women healers worked hard to comfort the sick and dying despite warnings from various church fathers and government officials that only licensed professionals could minister to the sick. It was during the 1300s that organized efforts by priests and male doctors to destroy women healers began.

Great upheaval continued in Europe even after the plague subsided in the late 1400s. The feudal system was being challenged by large peasant uprisings, many said to have been led by women. Protestant churches were gaining popularity, as were the ideas of capitalism. Women healers posed a serious threat to the economic security and patriarchal beliefs of the male medical professionals. Using women as scapegoats for natural disasters, for a man's impotency, for the sudden sickness or death of her neighbor's animals or family members, and for diseases that male doctors could not heal, were some of the ways priests and male doctors targeted women as the cause of all the suffering. Older women who were widowed and more dependent on their neighbors for support were accused of being witches, as were women who had never married. Women with little or no money were accused. Witchcraft persecution was also a method used for dealing with conflicts between neighbors.[2]

The burning and killing of several thousand women (the exact number is not known) from the fourteenth to the seventeenth century was conducted by the Catholic and Protestant churches and the male-dominated medical profession. Over 85 percent of the people accused of being witches were women.[3] Many of them were the unlicensed healers who were the primary health care providers for peasant people in villages across Europe.

Women of all ages, from various religious and class backgrounds, married and unmarried, were killed along with other targeted groups, such as lesbians, gay men, and Jews.

The gruesome executions were public events. Burning witches alive at the stake and hanging them in the public square was the common practice. Before being killed they were often forced to endure violent torture such as having unbearable pressure applied to their thumbnails and having their limbs stretched until they confessed something or named another witch. Thea Jensen, a feminist writer and broadcaster, calls the witch burnings the women's holocaust. They were a way to terrorize other women and children so that they would not deviate from the norm or show support to the already condemned.

The book *Malleus Maleficarum* was published by two Dominican priests in 1484. In it they explicitly explained how to conduct a witch-hunt. With the advent of the printing press, the book was mass produced. Witch-/heretic-hunts became well organized and many jobs were created, especially for lawyers and judges.

In England, the prevailing belief about witches was that they could do supernatural harm to others by using destructive spells, medicines, curses, and charms. Three different Witchcraft Acts were passed by Parliament. The first, in 1542, made the practice of witchcraft a statutory offense. The second act, passed in 1563, made evoking evil spirits illegal. The third act, passed in 1604, made any covenants with evil spirits a capital offense and also made it a felony to kill anyone by means of witchcraft.[4]

And witchcraft accusations did not end in 1736 when the Witchcraft Act of 1604 was repealed. Village people continued to believe in evil spirits and to blame witches for what they saw as supernatural occurrences. "Unauthorized" violence and occasional lynchings still occurred, as was evidenced by the hanging of a woman named Ruth Osborne in Hertfordshire, England, in 1751.[5]

I recently learned from a Dutch friend about a weighing station in a village called Oudewater in southern Holland. During the first quarter of the sixteenth century the Emperor and King of Spain, Charles V, who ruled the Holy Roman Empire of the German Nations, wanted to put an end to the witch-hunts. He came up with the idea of a weighing station as a way for women to prove that they were not witches. If a woman weighed more than a feather, which of course she did, then she could not fly and therefore was not a witch. She would receive a piece of paper that said how much she weighed and that Charles V had declared she was not a witch.

The witch craze gradually ended in Europe as the industrial revolution took hold, along with the spread of scientific ideas, which did not validate supernatural powers and magic. However, the witch-hunts had been successful at wiping out women healers and excluding women from studying medicine.

Witchcraft accusations also occurred throughout the New England colonies during the seventeenth century and continued even into the eighteenth century. Between 1647 and 1692, fourteen women and two men were killed by their town authorities for practicing witchcraft and others were jailed. In 1692, fourteen women and six men were executed in Salem, Massachusetts, for practicing witchcraft. Over 140 people were tried during the late summer of 1692 and several were jailed in some of the villages neighboring Salem.

The word *witch* has been associated with evil and the devil for over seven hundred years. The truth about witches as herbalists and healers, and witchcraft as a spiritual tradition, has been misrepresented and overlooked in most history books and classes. It was not until 1952 that the U.S. Congress passed a law recognizing Witchcraft as an organized religion and protecting witches from discrimination. Yet, despite legal protection, witches are still misunderstood by society at large and portrayed as evil and weird by the media. The healing traditions and spiritual roots of European-Americans date back to witchcraft and to prepatriarchal Goddess-worshipping cultures. We are fortunate to have writers like Starhawk, Z Budapest, Marija Gimbutas, Barbara Walker, Vicki Noble, Deirdre English, Barbara Ehrenreich, Margot Adler, Robert Graves, and Jeanne Achteberg and a film producer like Donna Read, all of whom have done extensive research on the ancient Goddess-worshipping times, the history of witchcraft, or modern day witches, herbalists, and healers.

HEALTH REFORM IN THE UNITED STATES

Throughout the 1700s male doctors used various "barbaric" methods: bloodletting, leeches, and treatment with toxic substances, to purge the body of disease. Finally, in the 1830s, an increasingly high number of middle-class women became dissatisfied with these horrific medical practices, and with the philosophy of allopathic doctors in general, and created the Popular Health Movement. Many of the strange medical practices began to disappear, thanks to these women, but the allopathic philosophy of ridding the body of disease remained, and is still the prevalent belief system of Western medicine today.

The women who founded the Popular Health Movement believed that health could be achieved through good nutrition, clean water and air, exercise, sunshine, and the use of herbs when needed. Mary Joe Nichols was one of the most active participants in the movement. She and others began to write about natural self-cures, hygiene and nutrition, and the important role women played in strengthening their families' health by being educated in the area of health. The start of an organized women's rights movement coincided with this progressive health movement, which supported women becoming physicians and spoke out about poor, working-class women's health and oppressive working conditions. The women who instigated health reforms during this time helped move women from the privacy of their homes out into the public arena and into the healing professions. Women's commitment to healing in a more public way had only just begun.

A New Hampshire farmer named Samuel Thomson, who learned about herbal remedies from a woman herbalist, created an herbal movement which began around the 1820s and was strong until about 1845. By 1839, three million people were using the information Thomson publicized.[6] Samuel encouraged women to become herbal doctors and even spoke on the importance of women doctoring each other instead of women going to male doctors.[7] However, the simple and effective ways in which the women herbalists of this time worked were rarely credited by the male practitioners who elaborated upon their remedies in later years.

Even before Thomson died in 1841, the movement had split. The Physio-Medical Institute, spearheaded by Alva Curtis, reorganized itself in 1841. Alva Curtis was determined to see medical schools, hospitals, and dispensaries based on herbal treatments be created. In 1843, The Eclectic Medical Institute was formed in Cincinnati, Ohio, which consisted of, as far as I can tell, primarily men, who were educated botanical practitioners using indigenous plants. In 1872 the National Eclectic Medical Association was formed, and in the 1880s approximately ten thousand people were practicing Eclectic-based medicine, primarily seeing working-class people.[8]

Another point I wish to raise here is that the Eclectics and other botanical practitioners received much of their knowledge about plants from Native American people, but gave little credit to their sources. The exploitation of indigenous peoples' knowledge and the destruction of their lands and communities occurred throughout the 1800s and has continued into the present. This is a difficult piece of history that Western herbalists tend to ignore.

The use of homeopathic preparations (remedies that stimulate a person or animal's life force so optimum health can be restored) should not be forgotten in this brief overview. Homeopathy became popular during the 1840s despite increasing hostility from allopathic doctors who viewed it as quackery. By the 1860s, over two-thirds of the homeopathic practitioners were women, and over ten thousand homeopaths were practicing. The homeopaths were primarily administering to people in the upper class. Unfortunately, there were rifts between homeopathic and herbal practitioners because many homeopaths believed their system was much more sophisticated than botanical medicine—an attitude that some homeopaths still have today.

Because of the decline in standardized medical education and the rise of homeopathic physicians, the allopathic doctors joined their forces and created the American Medical Association in 1848 as a way to have control over medical education and licensing. By the latter part of the 1800s, over seventy thousand allopathic doctors were practicing. Most of their clients were from the middle class.

During the second half of the nineteenth century various women healers established nursing as a profession, founded churches with a spiritual healing foundation such as the Christian Science church, and began training to be allopathic doctors. These women had to challenge the predominant myths that only men were intellectually and physically capable of doctoring to the sick. They also had to challenge the Victorian attitudes that a woman must be passive and subordinate. Women studying to be physicians often found themselves keeping their mouths shut if they wanted to survive in the male-dominated medical community.

The specialized field of women's medicine became the avenue many women physicians were able to receive training in because this field posed less of a threat to male physicians. During the 1870s and 1880s, some women's medical colleges were established. Through the fundraising efforts of feminists and medical educators most medical schools would be coed. Johns Hopkins University was endowed with $500,000 for the purpose of educating women physicians and began classes in 1893. Seventy-five percent of the other all-male medical schools quickly followed suit. Women soon made up 25–37 percent of the total enrollment in allopathic schools.[9] By the turn of the century only one women's medical college still existed.

It should be pointed out that most of the women striving to be physicians had such uphill battles to fight in making inroads into an old-boys club that they mainly stuck to allopathic principles of medicine. Women's writings were not published regularly, nor were the women who taught male physicians about their herbal cures well known or given much credit. I can only assume that village women continued to practice herbalism and homeopathy in their homes and communities out of necessity and choice, just as we are doing today.

At the turn of the century, male doctors began to complain that their salaries were decreasing due to women doctors. Medical colleges stopped taking women students. Not surprisingly, people of color and people with little access to money also had a difficult time being accepted into medical schools. Around this same time, the AMA (American Medical Association) established a Council on Medical Education to control how medical education was to proceed. The Carnegie Foundation hired Abraham Flexner, a schoolmaster who had no experience in medicine, to visit medical schools and determine which ones were following the AMA's guidelines and thus worthy of receiving money from foundations like Carnegie's. Flexner wrote a report in 1910 that drastically changed the course of medicine. He totally opposed any form of herbal, homeopathic, or holistic healing practice. The Flexner Report set the stage for the allopathic medical education model that still exists today.

The Eclectic and homeopathic medical schools operating at the turn of the century and offering training in botanical and homeopathic medicine began to close their doors. These schools were unable to compete with the allopathic schools, which were financially backed by the powerful upper class. New ideas about bacteria began to make herbal medicine look old-fashioned and it lost its popularity. John M. Scudder and John King, Eclectic doctors and visionaries, both died in the 1890s, and no other Eclectic visionaries followed them.[10]

The Lloyd Library in Cincinnati, Ohio, houses the majority of the Eclectic textbooks, some of which have been reprinted and are once again for sale. These books contain useful information on clinical application of herbs. Yet the Eclectic doctors were also mostly men. What were the contributions of the handful of women working within this system? And what successes were the laywomen healers having in their communities?

Since the early 1900s allopathic medicine has made huge advances with surgical technology and antibiotics, yet very little progress in changing its attitudes about meeting the needs of the whole person versus just treating symptoms. Today, only 17 percent of all allopathic physicians in the United States are women.[11] Over 80 percent of all medical care workers are women, yet they receive much lower wages and recognition than male doctors.[12] Women medical students are still often faced with hostility from male teachers and students that makes cultivating a more nurturing and compassionate approach to healing difficult. Fortunately, there are a growing number of naturopathic doctors, many of whom are women, being trained in botanical and homeopathic medicine today in Oregon, Washington, and Arizona. However, medical licensing varies from state to state, and at this point in time creates difficulties or limitations for some naturopathic doctors.

Women around the world, some of whom call themselves feminists, and some of whom may have never heard the word *feminist*, are beginning to recognize that the conventional, allopathic medical system's fundamental assumptions about women are oppressive and full of errors.

The Women's Health Movement began in the late 1960s in the United States as women joined together to reclaim knowledge about, and control over, their bodies and health care choices. This movement continues to grow around the world. Knowing the work of the women healers who went before us and the history of allopathic medicine, which excludes us, helps us unite to obtain quality health care today.

The hatred and fear of women and nature that spurred the European witch burnings still exists. Today's institutionalized oppressions—sexism, racism, homophobia, classism, and ageism—run rampant in all systems, including the allopathic and holistic medical systems, and are fed by a class system that still supports white male power. All of us, women and men both, have been deeply wounded by these oppressive belief systems. They wear out our bodies and spirits and in turn leave us unable to think about how to get the support we need to change our attitudes and actions. We often end up turning against ourselves and each other instead of joining together.

Today, as I sit finishing this book, the Food and Drug Administration is moving in the direction of classifying herbs as drugs and legally barring herbalists and manufacturers from making any claims on the therapeutic uses of them. It is more imperative than ever that we women keep the herbal tradition alive and figure out ways to support each other. It will take continuous work and honest soul-searching for us to create respectful relationships with each other that honor our diversity and place healing in the forefront of our daily preoccupations.

I hope that the herbal information in this book will be of help to any woman looking for practical, affordable, and nurturing ways to support herself, her family (including animal friends), and her community. Herbs, when used wisely and thoughtfully, keep us in balance with Earth and connected to the wise women who walked before us.

2

Creating an Herbal Apothecary

Sometimes when technological medicine has nothing more to offer a person, we may find the deepest healing in a simple green blossom.

—AMANDA McQUADE CRAWFORD

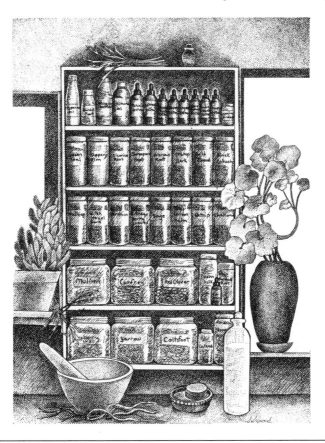

*H*aving my kitchen shelves filled with jars of dried herbs and bottles of tinctures and oils that I have made is deeply satisfying. The yearly gathering and drying of specific herbs connects me with nature's cyclical ways. Knowing which herbs to call upon for various health problems is reassuring to me. Turning to the herbs that grow in my garden and nearby fields and woods continuously delights me. Encouraging other women to grow and gather herbs and make and use them gives me hope that herbal healing will once again become accessible to all people. This chapter includes information on how to gather and dry herbs and how to make various types of herbal remedies. If the information given here is completely new to you, ask a friend to come join you and have fun exploring the world of herbs together.

GATHERING HERBS

When you approach a plant you wish to harvest, sit or kneel next to it. Quiet yourself by taking some deep breaths and allow yourself time to hear and feel life pulsing under and around you. Ask the plant if she will share her gifts with you. Let her know your intention—that you have come to ask for her medicine. When I was a teenager I was taught to look for the grandmother plant, the plant that looks larger, older, and more vibrant than the other plants, and to speak with her, make proper offerings to her, but never harvest her. Your gift of gratitude can be anything that feels close to your heart: a song, a prayer, or a piece of your hair. I like to bow to plants in the same way I bow during Buddhist ceremonies and meditations, deeply honoring the herb's presence and healing gifts.

Remember you are not alone as you gather herbs. Birds, butterflies, insects, plant devas, fairies and angels, and other animals may be nearby, sometimes visible and sometimes not. Move as slowly as you can. Collecting herbs offers us the opportunity to practice being mindful, attentive, and aware of how all life is interconnected. With this in mind, be sure to only collect wild plants that grow in abundance and harvest only what you need. Gather from areas where the plants are prolific and not threatened or endangered. Contact your area's wildflower society and state's conservation department for lists of endangered plants. You may want to join with other people who are helping to repopulate wild plants through proper propagation methods. (Always check out a nursery or mail-order business that sells wild plants to be sure they are not digging them from the wild.) Also, be absolutely sure you have identified any plant you harvest correctly. If in doubt, ask a local botanist or herbalist for verification before harvesting.

HARVESTING WITH THE MOON

Plants have specific times in their life cycles when their medicine is strongest. Certain roots are more potent when dug in the spring or fall because the plant is not busy producing leaves and flowers. The energy of roots is more concentrated at new moons and they are best when dug just before the new moon. Various calendars mark when the moon is full or new. Lunar calendars, which give guidance on planting and harvesting with the moon, are listed in the resource section.

Leaves, flowers, stems, twigs, and fruits are considered to be aboveground parts of plants and are best gathered between the new and full moons. Leaves and flowers are strongest when collected on clear, sunny days in the morning before the sun's rays have caused the plants to wilt. Wait until the dew has evaporated from the plants if your intention is to dry the leaves or flowers because it hinders the drying process. You will also want to collect them just after the full moon because their water content will be lower. If you wish to tincture the plants then you can pick them with dew just before the full moon. My friend Adele Dawson taught me that dew itself is healing and is a magical addition to your tincture.

Look for the leaves and flowers that feel vibrant and full of life energy. Avoid ones that are bruised, discolored, or full of insect holes. When gathering flowers, do so soon after they open. They are stronger before lots of bees frolic in their nectar.

Tree barks are best collected in the early spring when the buds are swelling, but before the leaves unfold, or in the fall as the leaves begin to drop from the trees and when the waning moon is in the third quarter. Prune branches from trees or shrubs that are crowding or entangling each other. Use a small pruning saw or shears. Then scrape the bark from these branches with a sharp pocketknife. This method ensures the tree's life will continue since you are not taking bark from the main trunk.

In the autumn I collect and save seeds from various plants growing in my gardens. Saving seeds is fun and also important since in many countries seed banks have been destroyed and non-hybrid varieties are being lost. (Refer to list of plant and seed resources in resource section for seed companies and seed-saving projects.) The ripening of seeds is different for every plant, and close observation is needed for collecting seeds at the right stage because seed heads will burst and the seeds will scatter if left too long. Collect the seeds in brown paper bags and then store in a cool place in glass jars or bags that are labeled with the seed's name and date harvested. Refer to books on seed propagation for specific planting information.

Baskets or clean brown paper bags work well for gathering herbs since both of these containers ensure good air circulation. Leave yourself plenty of time following harvesting to properly pre-pare the herbs into tinctures or teas or to lay them out on screens for drying. Freshly picked plants left lying around begin to lose their strength and vitality and can mold if left piled on top of each other, particularly leaves and flowers. Plants who give us their med-icine deserve our complete respect in return.

Drying Herbs

Drying herbs properly is as important as harvesting them. Be cre-ative with the spaces available to you for drying. Some basic guide-lines include a warm area with good air circulation like an attic, a stairwell, a ceiling where warm air rises, or above a wood stove. An ideal drying temperature is 85–100°F. Avoid using areas where direct sunlight would contact the plants for long periods of time since this will fade their color and lessen their potency. Use non-metal screens to dry herbs on. Take old screen frames and cut out the metal screening or make wooden frames and staple in fiberglass mesh, which is available at most hardware stores.

With experience, you will learn what specific plants feel like when dried correctly. When placing herbs on a screen, check them once or twice a day to see how the drying process is progressing. Herbs that are not dried enough will mold when stored away in glass jars. Herbs that are overdried will crumble when crushed between your fingers. Excess moisture in the air from rain or fog causes drying times to be longer.

We light the woodstove to drive out the dampness and cold during wet days here and have just purchased a dehumidifier to help get rid of excess moisture. A gas stove with a pilot light in the oven is also a good place for drying small amounts of herbs on cookie sheets, especially basil and parsley. Place the herbs on cookie sheets and leave them in the oven with the door cracked slightly. Make a big sign alerting yourself to take out the herbs before turning on the oven.

Store your dried herbs in glass jars or brown paper bags placed inside a sealed plastic bag. Label each jar or bag with the herb's name and date of harvest. Dried leaves and flowers hold their medicinal properties for a year and roots and tree barks for two years. Whatever dried herbs you have left over after a year or two can be put into a compost pile.

YOUR HERBAL MEDICINE CHEST

An herbal medicine chest lined with tincture bottles, flower essences, oils, and jars of dried herbs offers reassurance and hope to anyone in need. There are many ways to prepare herbal remedies, and each herbalist usually has her favorite methods. Use your intuition, knowledge, and skills and build upon your previous experiences when creating recipes and methods you like, and which work. Open your heart to the magic and surprises the plants offer.

TEAS

Preparing tea is an ancient ritual. It is a simple act that adds warmth and pleasure to women sharing their life stories over a steaming cup of tea. Herbal teas are used for administering both nourishment and medicine. The process of making tea directly connects us with the elements of water, fire, air, and the green gifts from Earth, helping realign us with the healing energies in nature.

A tea made by steeping or infusing leaves, flowers, and certain seeds—like fennel and anise, which are high in volatile oils—in hot, steaming water is called an infusion. Crumble or gently crush dried plants to open their cellular structures to the water. If you are using fresh leaves and flowers for your tea, you can either chop them or use them whole. I prefer to use them whole rather than chopping them in order to enjoy their beauty.

To make an infusion from dried herbs, place the herbs into a pint or quart glass jar or teapot. Use 1–3 teaspoons of dried herbs for every cup of water. Often I place 6 tablespoons of herbs into a glass quart jar in order to have a jar of tea to sip from throughout the day. Pour hot, steaming water over the herbs and let them steep, covered, five to ten minutes, or longer, for a stronger, more medicinal tea.

If you are using fresh herbs for your tea, use at least twice the amount you would use if the herb were dry. This is because the water content in fresh herbs dilutes their flavor. You do not have to be exact in your measurements. Let your hands, eyes, nose, and heart guide you. Place the fresh herbs into a glass, enamel, or stainless-steel pan, cover with cool water, and slowly bring the water to a simmer. Turn off the heat and steep, covered, for as long as you wish. Strain and enjoy your tea. On hot and humid summer days I add some unsweetened fruit juices to my fresh lemon balm and mint teas for a cooling and refreshing beverage.

Solar and Lunar Teas

The amount of chemical constituents and flavor extracted in a solar or lunar tea is less than for herbs infused in hot, steaming water. However, the sun's and moon's rays add their energy to teas as they infuse and offer special qualities only you will know.

To make sun tea: Place fresh or dried herbs into a glass jar, pour cool water over the herbs, and cover with a lid. Place in a hot, sunny location for several hours.

To make a moon tea: Gather fresh flowers and leaves, or use dried herbs, and place them in a clear glass bowl. Cover the herbs with cool water and leave the bowl uncovered in the full-moon light all night. You can also try making tea during different phases of the moon. Moon tea is full of subtle, mysterious, and magical qualities.

Decoctions

A decoction is a tea made with hard or woody parts of herbs such as roots, tree barks, and different seeds and nuts. Place 4–6 tablespoons of dried herb pieces into a glass, enamel, or stainless-steel pan and cover with a quart of cool water. Let sit overnight and then slowly bring to a boil and simmer, covered, for twenty to thirty minutes. If you do not have the time to steep the herbs overnight, you can simmer the herbs an additional ten to twenty minutes. Strain and save the herbs for one more batch of tea. The second batch of tea usually has less flavor, but there are still health-promoting properties to receive. Add some new herbs to the already used ones if you want a stronger flavor. Drink your tea throughout the day. If you have some left at the end of the day, store it in the refrigerator and slowly reheat it on the stove the next day before drinking.

TINCTURES

Tinctures are usually alcohol- and water-based preparations, although today there are some tinctures made from glycerine on the market. Glycerine, a sweet, mucilaginous liquid, is an effective solvent for only certain herbs. It is useful for children or people who cannot tolerate any alcohol. Some people also use vinegar to make tinctures, though vinegar is not a very strong solvent for extracting medicinal properties into solution.

Alcohol is more commonly used because it easily extracts alkaloids, resins, and volatile oils while vinegar only extracts alkaloids and minerals and vitamins. Glycerine extracts similar chemical constituents to alcohol, but not as strongly as alcohol.

Many herb companies use 190-proof grain alcohol because it allows them to be much more specific with the percentages of alcohol to water that they use for each individual herb. For home purposes however, 100-proof vodka (some people prefer brandy) works fine.

Alcohol, glycerine, and vinegar act as preservatives and tinctures therefore have a longer shelf life than dried herbs. Some herbalists say alcohol tinctures last for at least ten years. Glycerines need to be stored in the refrigerator and may last up to a year. The shelf life of vinegars may vary depending on the quality and percentage of acetic acid of the vinegar. If any of these liquid extracts go bad they will smell funky and moldy.

Herbs ingested in tincture form are quickly absorbed into the bloodstream. Tinctures are easy to travel with and to administer in first aid situations. They are useful when someone is in bed with a flu or broken bone and cannot make tea, but can still reach for the tincture bottle. Tinctures are also convenient for people caretaking children, elderly people, and animals. Another advantage of tinctures is that they allow someone to ingest an herb that they might otherwise not be able to because of the herb's extremely bitter or otherwise unpalatable taste. Tinctures are also a method of preserving herbs that can only be used when fresh.

The amount of tincture drops taken internally depends on body weight and the severity of the situation being treated. A simple guideline to follow is one to two drops of tincture for five pounds of body weight. Place the drops in a small cup of water or juice or directly into an animal's food. A 25-pound child or dog would get 5–10 drops and a 125-pound adult or goat would get 25–50 drops. Nursing infants can receive the herb's properties through their mother's milk.

The amount of times a tincture is taken daily depends on the situation you are working with. For nourishing and restoring strength and tone to a particular organ, like the liver, a tincture is taken three to four times per day for one to two months, or longer if needed. Give smaller amounts more frequently for an acute illness every half hour. To avoid alcohol, place the drops in boiling water, remove from the stove, and wait a few minutes before administering. A large percentage of the alcohol will have evaporated. People who are recovering alcoholics, or who are extremely sensitive to alcohol, may choose to use this method, or may want to completely avoid using alcohol tinctures. The hot water method is a good one to use when giving tinctures to children and animals.

Throughout the book, under each formula, I list different herbs to use in combination. After each herb is listed how many parts to use when mixing together the different herbal tinctures. For example, the liver tonic formula listed in chapter 5 looks like this:

Dandelion roots—2 parts

Milk thistle seed—2 parts

Blessed thistle—1 part

Chicory root—1 part

Wild yam root—2 parts

You can use whatever measurement you want for parts as long as you are consistent with what you use. You can let 1 part equal 1 teaspoon or 1 tablespoon, or, if you are mixing a quart jar of a particular formula, you can let the 1-part measurement be ⅛ of a cup. These guidelines are the same when making tea.

Preparing a Tincture From Fresh Plants

Tinctures are simple and fun to make. When made mindfully and with good quality herbs they contain strong medicine. Fresh plants embody the vital life force (contained within all plants) and I believe this vital life force adds to a tincture's potency.

There are many ways to prepare tinctures. The following directions are basic guidelines to assist those of you who have never made tinctures.

- After carefully harvesting the plants you need, check them over and compost damaged parts of the plants, such as rotten sections of a root, or yellow or chewed leaf tips.

- Wash leaves and roots if they are muddy.

- Fill a glass jar full of plant matter, leaving an inch of space. (I prefer to tincture each herb separately and mix combinations as I need them.) Completely cover plants with 100-proof vodka, brandy, or vinegar and secure the lid tightly. Shake the bottle fifty to one hundred times. Offer a prayer or song if you wish. I also like to bow to each freshly made tincture.

- Label and date each tincture. Include the name of the plant and the part used. You might want to record your measurements in a recipe book. Also include the place you harvested from and any interesting weather information or observations you made. I enjoy looking back year after year and seeing what the weather was like or what bird I saw when harvesting.

- Place jars in a dark closet or cupboard and let sit for two to six weeks. Shake your bottle every day. During the first week of extraction, you may need to top off your jar as the plants absorb liquid. This ensures the plants will stay completely covered in liquid (called menstrum) while tincturing.

- After two to six weeks, strain the tincture through cheesecloth. An easy way to do this is to place a stainless-steel colander in a large bowl and pour the liquid into the cheesecloth. Tightly wring the cheesecloth, which contains the plant matter, to get out what extra liquid you can. At Avena we have a large stainless-steel press that exerts eight tons of pressure on the herbs wrapped in an unbleached cotton cloth. For home purposes, cheesecloth is sufficient unless you want to purchase a small wine press or make a press with a hydraulic jack.

- Pour all your liquid into a glass bottle with a tight-fitting lid. Label and date your tincture and store in a dark, cool place.

Preparing a Tincture From Dried Plants

Some people only have access to dried plants, and a few plants, such as blue cohosh, are better tinctured from the dried roots.

- Take 4 ounces of dried herbs and grind to a powder in a good quality coffee grinder or blender.

- Place the herbs into a 1-pint glass jar and fill the jar to the top with vodka, or brandy, and secure lid tightly. Complete your tincture using the same instructions as the fresh tincture procedures.

Glycerine Tincture

Glycerine is a sweetish, mucilaginous, thick liquid derived from plant or animal sources. One hundred percent vegetable glycerine is available through herb stores and health food stores, though you may need to have it specially ordered. Glycerine is able to extract plant alkaloids* along with the mucilage found in some plants, such as marshmallow and comfrey roots, but does not extract the resin type substance such as that found in balm of gilead buds.

Different herbalists use different proportions of water and glycerine depending on whether they are using fresh plants (you would use only glycerine) or dried plants. Experiment with what you like. The following guidelines are for dried plants.

- Powder 4 ounces of herbs. Place in a pint glass jar. Mix 1½ cups of vegetable glycerine and ½ cup of distilled water together and pour over herbs. Secure lid tightly. Follow directions under fresh tinctures for completing the process.

HERBAL VINEGARS

I prefer to use a good quality organic apple cider vinegar or brown rice vinegar for making delicious and nutritious herbal vinegars to use on salads, in soups, and in sauces. Use the various culinary herbs such as tarragon, basil, rosemary, and thyme and a touch of the spring tonic greens such as dandelion, chickweed, and nettle. Fill a glass jar with fresh herbs and cover with vinegar. Cap with a glass or plastic lid and place in the direct sunlight. Separate the vinegar from the herbs after four to six weeks by pouring through cheesecloth. Store in a glass jar with a glass or plastic lid in a dark, cool cupboard.

FLOWER ESSENCES

Every living flower contains its own unique vibrational pattern. A flower essence embodies this vibrational pattern by sun-infusing flowers in spring water for four to eight hours. Flower essences act as catalysts to reawaken the natural life force within us. They support our abilities to transform limiting emotions, behaviors, and attitudes into more health-affirming ways of living and being. Flower essences are taken orally under the tongue, four drops at a time, or placed onto the skin, as many times a day as you wish.

---

*Herbs contain a variety of chemical constituents, alkaloids and mucilages being two kinds.

They can also be very helpful for animals and are administered by placing drops in their water dishes, letting them lick drops directly off your hand, or placing the drops directly on their heads. This last way is easy to do with injured wild animals.

Flower essences were rediscovered in the 1930s by a physician, Dr. Edward Bach, in England. Dr. Bach spent four years meditating with different English flowers and created thirty-eight flower essences, which he named the Bach Flower Essences. They are available in many health food stores and through mail-order catalogs.

In the late 1970s a small group of health practitioners in California began researching and preparing flower essences from California flowers. They now call themselves the Flower Essence Service and offer several hundred flower essences, many excellent books, and training courses. Since that time other people have begun making flower essences from their local areas including Woodland Essences, which focus on flowers from trees, and Flowers of the Soul, which support soul transformation. I have also prepared dozens of flower essences from my gardens and have found them to be particularly useful for animals.

How to Make Flower Essences

Keep a few small clear glass bowls and tiny flower clippers set aside for making flower essences. Pour boiling water over the clippers and glass bowl to sterilize them before using them.

On a clear, sunny morning, go to the flower you wish to make an essence from. Spend time sitting with the flower and feel or listen for the flower's message to you. If this is new for you, practice sitting quietly with various flowers on a regular basis.

Carefully hold the bowl filled with room/air temperature spring water under the flowers you are gathering. I was taught to cut each flower without touching it with my fingers and let it fall into the spring water. Fill the bowl full of flowers and then place it uncovered on the earth near the plants you were collecting from. The sun's energy will infuse the flower's vibrations into the water. Let the wise woman in you guide you as to the length of time the flowers want to be infusing in the spring water. Some may be for a

few hours and others may want to infuse
for a twenty-four-hour cycle. You may feel
drawn to make a flower essence in
the full-moon light or at specific
seasonal transitions like the
summer equinox.

When the
infusion process
is completed, take
the flowers out of
the water using the
clippers or a small
plant stem. Offer
some of the infused
spring water to the
plants the flowers
came from. Fill an
amber-colored,
sterilized glass
jar halfway with
the essence. Add the
same amount of brandy that
has been aged in oak (look on the label) as the amount of spring
water in the jar for preservation purposes. Label and date this
flower essence, which flower essence practitioners call the Mother
Essence. This is the bottle used to make further dilutions, which is
explained below. Store your essences in a special basket or place in
your house. Some people like to place various crystals and stones
near them.

Diluting Flower Essences

To make a stock bottle: Take 7 drops of the Mother Essence with
a sterilized glass dropper and add to a clean ¼-, ½- or 1-ounce
amber glass dropper bottle that contains half spring water and half
brandy. Label and store properly. Stock bottles are used to make the
personal remedy bottle, which is the dilution taken by a person or
animal.

To make a personal remedy bottle: Take 2–7 drops from each different stock flower essence bottle you wish to use and add to a sterilized 1-ounce amber glass dropper bottle that is nearly filled with spring water. Add 2 teaspoons of brandy, glycerine, or apple cider vinegar to the bottle as a preservative to prevent algae from growing. Tap the bottom of the bottle with your fingers 50–100 times to awaken the life force of the flower essence.

The way I was taught to choose which different flower essences were needed for a particular person or animal was by dowsing with a small pendulum. Some people use kinesiology, also called muscle testing. Some choose by reading the various descriptions written about certain flowers, and others intuit which essences are most needed. A flower essence can be used alone or in combination with other flower essences for as many days as the person feels drawn to take the essence. There is no one specific way to take a flower essence. You may find yourself taking less and less of the essence or forgetting to take it, which usually means you no longer need this specific flower essence. Because flower essences contain only the energy of the flower and no plant chemical constituents, you do not have to worry about any side effects and they are safe for pregnant and nursing women, infants, children, animals, and adults of all ages. In fact, young children usually like to touch and hold various bottles and watch the drops being placed into a bottle. They often enjoy being around magical and energy-charged spaces.

HERB-INFUSED OILS

There are many different approaches to making infused oils. Herb oils can be made with a variety of cold-pressed oils. Olive, safflower, sunflower, almond, apricot kernel, and sesame oil are some of the more commonly used oils. Avoid mineral oil, as it is petroleum based. I prefer to use organic olive oil since it is readily absorbed into the skin and does not go rancid as quickly as other oils. Organic olive oil is now available in many food co-ops and natural food stores.

Infused oils can be made from fresh and dried herbs. St.-Johnswort flowers, mullein flowers, and rue leaves are most effective when used fresh. Some people prefer to use calendula flowers fresh and others use the dried flowers. A good quality and organic comfrey root that is dried makes a nice oil. I have made arnica oil from both fresh and freshly dried plants and find them both equally useful. My favorite oil for curing ringworm in animals is fresh plantain oil mixed with calendula oil.

To Make Fresh Herb Oils

Fill a clean, dry glass jar to the top with fresh herbs. Slowly cover with oil. Use a knife or clean wooden chopstick to release the air between the herbs so they become fully surrounded by oil. If the jar is not filled to the top with oil, mold can grow in the open space. If this happens, remove the mold with a spoon and add a bit more oil to the jar. I use cheesecloth to cover the jar. Place the jar in a warm place that is not above 100°F, such as a gas oven with a pilot light, near a hot water heater, or in a sunny window. Keep an eye on the oil each day to ensure no mold is developing. After two weeks, separate the plant matter from the oil by pouring the oil from the jar through clean cheesecloth into another glass jar. Compost the plant matter. Cover the new jar with cheesecloth and let it sit undisturbed for one day. The water and sludge from the fresh plants that mixed with the oil during the infusion process will settle to the bottom of the jar. Carefully use a turkey baster to siphon off the oil that sits on top of the water and sludge and place in a clean glass jar. You may need to siphon the oil a few times before there is no more water present at the bottom. This method helps prevent your fresh oils from fermenting. Once your oil is free of water, place a tight-fitting lid on the jar and store in a dark, cool place.

To Make Dry Herb Oils

When using dried herbs to make an oil I use 2 parts oil to 1 part herb. If I wanted to make a pint of calendula oil I would place 2 cups of olive oil and 1 cup of dried calendula flowers into a blender and grind them together and then pour the mixture into a clean glass pint jar and cover with a lid and put in a warm place for two to four weeks. At the end of the infusing period I would pour off the oil through cheesecloth and press the remaining plant matter through Avena's press. For home purposes squeeze as much oil as you can out of the flowers using cheesecloth or a small press.

Bottle the oil, label and date it, and store in a dark, cool place. Most oils have a shelf life of one year.

Many different herbs can be made into oils. Some commonly used dried herbs include comfrey leaves and roots, calendula flowers, goldenseal roots, echinacea roots, mugwort flowers and leaves, borage leaves, red clover, and usnea. Some of the herbs I use fresh include plantain leaves, mullein flowers, yarrow flowers, rosemary, garlic, rue, St. Johnswort flowers and buds, witch hazel, and heartsease pansy. The different herbs chosen depend on the purpose for the oil. Herb oils help heal cuts, chapped lips, skin rashes, cracked and dry skin, hemorrhoids, inflammations, diaper rashes, and more.

SALVES

Salves are easy to make from herb-infused oils. I hope that someday herbal salves will be in all drugstores, hospitals, and veterinarian clinics. I created an herbal salve called Heal-All Salve in 1985 and I have never changed the recipe because it has helped hundreds of people and animals. Salves are full of strong green healing and are lots of fun to make. They heal cuts, abrasions, cracked and dry skin, chapped lips, hemorrhoids, diaper rashes, and more.

To make 8 ounces of salve, place 1 cup of herb-infused oil into a glass or enamel pot. Add 2 ounces of beeswax into the oil and slowly warm on the stove, stirring occasionally. Beeswax melts at 140°F and your goal is to melt the beeswax and have it thoroughly mixed in the herb oil. After this occurs, pour the warm liquid into small containers and watch the salve solidify before your eyes as the mixture cools. Magic. If you want a harder consistency to your salve, add a bit more beeswax. For a softer salve, add more oil. You can make smaller or larger amounts of salve by adjusting the proportions given above. Watch out—when your friends and neighbors find out you make salve they will be knocking at your door. Write down your recipes. You will want to know how to repeat the salve formula you really like.

HERB POULTICE

A poultice is made from either fresh or dried herbs. Freshly bruised herbs can be applied directly to the injury or placed between thin cotton cloth or gauze and then applied. A freshly picked and chewed plantain leaf applied directly onto a mosquito bite or bee sting is an excellent example of a poultice. Plantain brings the swelling down immediately, eases pain, and stops any bleeding.

When using dried herbs, make a paste by adding a small amount of hot herbal tea, hot apple cider vinegar, and/or 10–30 drops of tincture (or more for a larger poultice) to the amount of powdered herb needed for the area you are covering. If you have whole or cut roots, simmer them for twenty minutes in a small amount of water, just enough to soften them. Add some flour or marshmallow-root powder if the herb mash is too liquidy. This herbal mash can be placed between thin cloth and applied to the injury. Leave in place for ten to twenty minutes for minor first aid situations like bee stings or cuts and then compost the herbs.

For situations like arthritis, muscle spasms, swollen glands, abscesses, and sinus or bronchial congestion, keep the poultice moist and warm by covering with plastic and then a towel and a hot water bottle and leaving in place overnight or for thirty-minute periods a few times a day. These herbs will need to be composted and a new poultice applied each time.

HERB COMPRESS

A compress, sometimes referred to as a fomentation, is made by soaking a clean cotton cloth, such as a washcloth, in 3–4 cups of a hot herbal tea for five minutes. Carefully lift the hot cloth out of the tea with a pair of tongs, wring well with your hands once it is cool enough to touch, and place onto an area (or several areas, with as many cloths as needed) that is cold, inflamed, painful, or congested. Cover with a towel and a hot water bottle and then another towel to keep everything warm and leave in place for twenty to thirty minutes. Reapply with a new hot cloth if desired.

CASTOR-OIL PACK

Castor-oil packs are indicated for non-malignant cysts and uterine fibroids. They also help to detoxify specific organs such as the liver, improve circulation to a congested, weakened, or cold area, and relieve constipation, gall bladder inflammation and lymphatic congestion. You can buy good quality castor oil from a natural foods store. It is also available through drugstores, though the quality may not be as good.

Castor-oil packs are easy to do, yet a bit greasy because the oil is thick. Warm a small amount of castor oil in a glass or enamel pan. Place a soft cotton or wool flannel cloth into the oil and let it soak up the oil completely. Put the warm cloth over the growth or area needing assistance. Cover the cloth with plastic and then a towel and a hot water bottle. *Note:* It is important to eliminate the hot water bottle in the following situations: pregnancy, stomach ulceration, heavy menstrual flow and acute inflammations. I wear an old shirt and lie on a few old towels to avoid getting my sheets and other clothes stained with castor oil. Keep the hot water bottle on for at least an hour. Many health care providers recommend leaving the castor-oil pack, plastic, and towels on overnight. Wash your skin after taking off the pack with ½ teaspoon of baking soda mixed in ½ cup of water. Apply the pack three to five nights in a row, break for three days, and keep repeating until the situation has healed. You can wrap your oily cloth in plastic and store it in the refrigerator after each use. Use the same cloth for up to six weeks, adding a small amount of oil as needed to keep it moist. Remember to use your pack only on yourself.

BATHS

Foot, hand, full body, and sitz baths are healing and rejuvenating to the body. Baths stimulate circulation to a congested, cold, or crampy area of the body, move stagnant blood, relax and calm the body, break a fever, produce a sweat, detoxify the body, warm the body, and ease aches and pain.

Various herbs can be made into tea and then poured into a bath. Throughout this book certain herbal teas and essential oils are recommended for specific conditions.

A ginger bath is an easy and stimulating bath for the whole body or for just the hands or feet. Grate 4 tablespoons of fresh ginger root and steep in 1 quart of hot water for fifteen minutes and pour into a pan and soak cold, numb, or swollen hands for ten to fifteen minutes. Add more hot water if needed to maintain constant temperature.

For a foot bath, grate 8 tablespoons of ginger root and steep in

2 quarts of hot water for fifteen minutes. Pour into a pan large enough for your feet. Add enough hot water to cover feet and soak as long as you want, adding hot water to maintain constant temperature. This wonderful foot bath warms the whole body, improves circulation to the feet, eases mental tiredness, and soothes achy feet.

A hot ginger foot bath can also cause the body to sweat and a fever to be lowered. Be sure to completely wrap your body and head in a warm blanket, which should also surround the tub of steaming ginger tea. Stay seated for at least another five minutes after sweating begins, then quickly jump in a warm shower or rinse off the sweat in a warm room, put on clean, dry clothes, and get under lots of warm blankets and go to sleep.

A full body ginger bath improves overall circulation; eases achy joints, muscles, and bones; and warms the entire body. Grate 8–16 tablespoons of fresh root, add to a gallon of hot water, steep for fifteen minutes, strain, and pour into your bathwater and soak away.

Sitz Bath

Sitz baths improve circulation to the pelvic area. Herbal teas made with ginger root and prickly ash bark especially help stimulate circulation. Fill a shallow container, large enough to get your bottom and hips into, with 2–4 quarts of hot herbal tea and enough extra hot water to come up to your hips. Have another pan next to you with cold water. Sit in the hot water for five minutes and then in the cold water for one to two minutes. Alternate back and forth three or four times, adding hot and cold water to each pan to keep the temperatures constant. Do this four to five nights in a row, take a break for a few nights, and repeat as long as needed.

Herbal teas made with comfrey leaves, goldenseal root, and plantain are often recommended by midwives to add to a pan of warm water to help ease swelling, pain, and to heal perineum tissue (between the anus and vagina) tears after birth. Sit in this bath for ten to fifteen minutes a few times a day until soreness and inflammation have disappeared.

CLAY PASTE

Clay is a soil type and is alive. It contains life-giving and health-restoring properties. Clay varies in color depending upon what geographical area it is collected from. Green clay is often used for facials, and bentonite clay, which is white, is used for pulling out imbedded particles in the skin and drying up acne. Different kinds of clay powders are available through health food stores and herb companies.

Place whatever amount of clay you want into a clean glass jar. You can add a teaspoon of dried and powdered herbs or a few drops of herbal tincture depending on what you will use the clay for. Cover the clay with nonchlorinated water until it is an inch above the powdered clay. Let the water mix with the clay without mechanically stirring it. This avoids lumps. Clay paste stays moist and usable for three to four weeks if stored covered and in a dark place.

FACE STEAMS

Experiencing an herbal face steam is pure delight and cleansing to the skin. Make an herbal tea with any of the following herbs or others you prefer following directions listed earlier under teas: calendula flowers, chamomile, roses, lavender, comfrey leaves, lemon balm, sage, peppermint, or mugwort. Warm 1–2 quarts of the tea on the stove. Place your face over the steam so it feels inviting and not too hot. Cover your head and the pot with a towel so the steam will touch your face. Keep your head under the towel for as long as you like. Then cover your face with a clay paste. The clay helps draw out dirt. Leave the paste on for ten to fifteen minutes. The clay will begin to dry on your face and you can wash it off with warm water. Then cover your face with honey and leave that on for ten minutes. Wash it off with warm water. Honey is a wonderful skin moisturizer and leaves your whole face feeling refreshed, reenergized, and glowing. Invite some other women to join you and have fun.

3

Daily Teas and Edible Greens

Experience is our way back home
This work requires an unguarded heart
Improvising each day
Protect and celebrate a love that is wild
Throw flowers at all that is evil
There is magic among us
The source of our power is in the Earth
The birds teach us how to listen.

—TERRY TEMPEST WILLIAMS

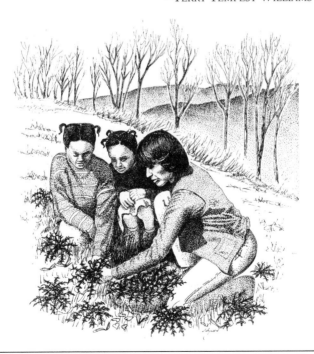

*I*n the spring and summer I am often out the door before 6 A.M., excited by the choruses of songbirds that fill the air and eager to see what new plant is up or flowering. I enjoy looking at the centers of flowers and leaves laden with the morning dew, sparkling as the sun's first rays creep down over the hillside and awaken them.

One morning I was standing still, watching the mist and listening to the dawn, when I heard a rufous-sided towhee call out "Drink your teeeee, drink your teeeeeee." I started laughing as I remembered my hot cup of tea sitting on the table.

If drinking tea made from organic or wild herbs is new for you, start with a few herbs. Use one at a time so you can learn to distinguish each herb's unique flavor. You will be in for delightful surprises if you are accustomed to drinking commercial-grade teas. The freshness and vitality can be tasted in herbs that are grown without chemicals and gathered and prepared thoughtfully.

If you grow or gather herbs from the wild, sit quietly with them before harvesting. Gently hold your hands near, yet not touching, and begin to feel the life energy pulsing from them. Let the plants know why you have come, ask their permission before harvesting, leave an offering such as a prayer, a special herb, a song, or a piece of your hair in return for their gifts. Take only what you need, being sure to leave plenty for the plant's continued survival and for other gatherers.

Here are a handful of my favorite nourishing herbs. Some are safe to use on a daily basis over several months; others are better to use a few times a week or during seasonal changes. Nourishing herbs replenish the health and vitality of the body by supporting the body's inherent metabolic processes of strengthening, toning, and rebuilding. Some of the nourishing herbs listed elsewhere also help to regulate and balance the hormonal system because of their specific chemical constituents. Included in this chapter is information on how to grow, collect, prepare, and use the herbs described.

44

ALFALFA   (*Medicago sativa*) *Leguminosae*, Pea Family
Other common names: Lucerne, Purple medic, Spanish clover
Parts used: Leaves and flowers

Alfalfa is a deep-rooted legume with beautiful violet-blue flowers. The leaves are pinnate, with three denticulate leaflets that grow up to three centimeters long. The stalks can grow to be over six feet high with many branching stems. The genus *Medicago* comes from Medea, in North Africa, which is where some botanists say alfalfa originated. The species *sativa* means cultivated.

Fields of alfalfa are often planted in the Northeast for hay or as a cover crop. Alfalfa enriches the soil because of its ability to fix nitrogen. Several years ago I was running in some woods in Concord, Massachusetts, and came out into a field planted with alfalfa that was over five feet high. I loved running through the alfalfa, feeling it gently brush against my skin, smelling its sweet scent.

Alfalfa is a perennial and is harvested in midsummer when the plant is in full bloom. Cut the stalks, bunch them, and hang them to dry. Once the hanging bunches are dry, strip the leaves and flowers from the stems and store them in a tightly sealed glass jar.

Alfalfa tea, made from fresh or dried leaves and flowers, is nourishing to the body because it contains carotene and chlorophyll[1] and other useful vitamins and minerals. Alfalfa tea helps regulate the stomach's pH level and is useful for people with hyperacidic stomachs to drink twenty minutes before eating, several times a week. People who eat lots of carbohydrates may also find their digestive systems work better when they drink a cup of alfalfa tea four to five times per week.

Alfalfa helps saliva to be secreted, which begins the early breakdown of starches in the mouth, thereby increasing appetite and encouraging weight gain. Alfalfa tea is of great benefit for anyone who has lost blood or is anemic to drink for several weeks. Some midwives recommend alfalfa tea be taken on a daily basis throughout pregnancy because of its high nutrient content and to prevent excessive hemorrhaging after birth. Alfalfa can be mixed with other herbs, such as peppermint, spearmint, fennel seed, catnip, and chamomile flowers and made into a tea for easing stomachaches or just for adding interesting flavors. Alfalfa tea is also nutritionally supportive for women experiencing menopause.

Fresh alfalfa leaves and flowers are a delightful addition to a green salad, as are alfalfa sprouts. Alfalfa is still widely cultivated for animal fodder in many countries and several different varieties are available.

Steep fresh or dried alfalfa leaves and flowers, covered, in hot, steaming water for ten to thirty minutes, and drink 1 cup of tea, warm or cool, twenty minutes before meals, or as needed.

CALENDULA   (*Calendula officinalis*) *Compositae*, Daisy Family
Other common names: Pot marigold (calendula
   is not a true marigold), marigold, sun
   flower, Mary bud
Part used: Flower, yellow and orange

Calendula is one of my favorite garden
herbs. I always smile when I come upon a
patch of flowering calendulas. Their brilliant
colors bring a feeling of joy to my heart. Each
flower's center is a unique mandala filled
with delicate miniature flowers that outline
the center like a wreath a fairy might wear.
Every flower has its own special characteris-
tics and I easily become absorbed in noticing
this when harvesting them.

Calendula

Calendula is an annual that can grow to two feet high if the soil is rich in organic matter. The leaves are smooth, oblong, and three to six inches long. The flower heads are two to four inches across and are borne on a beautifully crown-shaped receptacle. The petals drop off as the flower begins to die and a circular corona of seeds is left. Some people comment on how much the seeds look like curly worms.

Once a calendula bed or path is established in your garden there will always be some plants returning because of how easily calendula reseeds itself. Scatter seeds or plant them in rows in the fall or early spring. In Maine, we direct seed from late April until mid-May. If you start seedlings indoors or buy them, wait until the threat of frost is over before planting them outside. These plants do give earlier blooms to the northern gardener who is hungry for flowers.

In my labyrinth-shaped herb garden, four large calendula beds wind around the center mound, offering many pounds of flowers each summer. Calendula plants keep blooming if the flowers are picked every few days. From mid-July until mid-September I am out in the calendula gardens gathering the blossoms as they first begin to open. Your fingers will feel sticky after picking the flowers. This is from the flowers' resin, which is revered for healing cuts and wounds. Flowers harvested before they have fully opened contain higher amounts of resin.

On sunny days, once the dew has left the flowers, harvest calendula flowers into baskets. Be careful to limit how many flowers you place on top of each other. Flowers sweat when crowded together. This extra wetness hinders the drying process. Lay the flowers onto screens as soon as you have finished gathering. They take longer to dry than other herbs because of the thickness of their center. Flowers that are not fully dried will mold if placed in glass jars. Test their dryness by feeling their centers. Take them from the screens and store whole in glass jars when the centers are completely dry.

Calendula flowers offer many healing gifts. Each summer I make a few gallons of fresh calendula tincture, but mostly I dry the flowers for teas, salves, oils, and for feeding my animal friends.

Calendula can be used internally and externally for various ailments. Taken internally as a tea or tincture, calendula helps reduce swollen glands and is a safe herb for children and adults to take during measles and chicken pox along with other herbs. It is a useful herb to take for indigestion, helps heal gastric and duodenal ulcers when used over several weeks in combination with other herbs, and offers some relief for gallbladder problems.

A strong infusion or diluted tincture of calendula makes an excellent antiseptic wash for any wound, burn, skin infection, rash, herpes sores, eczema, or skin that is itchy, dry, and flaky. Use the tea or diluted tincture as a mouth rinse for inflamed or infected gums and as an eye wash for infected, scratched, or irritated eyes.

Calendula flowers are an excellent addition to any salve or oil. Topically, they heal cuts, burns, dry skin, chapped lips, infected and inflamed wounds, skin ulcers, and slow-to-heal cuts. Use a calendula oil or salve to prevent scarring after a wound with stitches is dry and during the final stages of poison ivy or chicken pox. Do be aware that a wound with stitches will heal more quickly when a calendula salve is used. If the stitches are ones that need to be removed, take care to watch the healing process closely as the stitches will most likely need to come out earlier than the doctor thinks.

The heal-all salve I created years ago for Avena Botanicals, which contains calendula and other herbs, has been an amazing salve for hundreds of people and animals. It has proved to be especially healing for women who have radiation burns on their breasts, and I can report specific cases where it helped make for the quick healing of a man who sustained a deep, gashing wound when a transformer box tore open the side of his face, and for a woman carpenter whose work partner had put a nail through two of her fingers with an electric nail gun. It also expedited the healing of a bird with an injured wing. Herbs grown and prepared properly are deeply healing. Creating your own salve recipes is fun and rewarding.

Calendula salve, oil, or tea is effective for relieving various skin irritations that itch. Calendula and plantain oils are effective in eliminating ringworm. For stubborn cases of ringworm or other skin funguses, apply undiluted ti tree oil directly onto infected areas and then apply calendula and plantain oil. This works well for people and animals.

Calendula oil is wonderful to rub into dry, cracked feet and hands. Every spring my hands feel extremely dry when I begin full-time gardening. Daily applications of a calendula salve alleviate this problem.

My dog Mochi loves to eat calendula salve off my fingers. Don't hesitate to mix calendula tea, tincture, oil, or a teaspoon of dried and powdered flowers into any animal's food, especially if they have dry skin or are constantly itching. Apply salve or oil onto their wounds or areas that are dry and irritated. Many people call during flea season when their dogs are itching and chewing their backs raw. Rinsing the area every day with calendula, red clover, and nettle tea and applying a calendula salve heals these hot spots.

If you have only a small garden plot, calendula is an herb to consider growing because of its beauty and many beneficial uses. I add a few teaspoons of the dried flowers to my teapot, four or five days a week, throughout the fall and winter. Calendula flowers add bright colors to a winter tea and are fun to watch reconstitute as they steep in your teapot. The flowers appear whole and alive as if they had been recently picked. In the depths of winter and snow, calendula flowers offer sunshine and hope that the coming gardening season will arrive.

CHAMOMILE (*Anthemis nobilis*) (perennial) and (*Matricaria recutita*) (annual) *Compositae*, Daisy Family
Other common names: Ground apple
Part used: Flowers and leaves

In Maine, chamomile can be planted soon after planting peas, mid to late April, and throughout May, by scattering seeds and gently pressing them into the soil with your hand or the back of a hoe, or lightly scratching the soil with the back of a rake. The center of this tiny, daisylike flower is yellow with ten or more white ray flowers surrounding it. The stalks are very thin, growing up to two feet, and the leaf segments are delicate and finely divided. Annual chamomile, also known as German chamomile, originated in Europe and western Asia.[2]

The annual chamomile reseeds itself year after year. Every few years I mix in a small amount of compost and scatter some extra seeds and the flowers continue to be luscious and sweet smelling. I leave a path next to the chamomile beds wide enough for me and my dog Mochi to lie in. When the chamomile is blooming, which it does for several weeks each midsummer, we take naps together in a special spot, breathing in the wonderful fragrance and enjoying each other's company.

Chamomile tea is a common remedy for a wide range of health conditions. It is a favorite bedtime tea for children and adults, soothing, relaxing, and calming to the body. Chamomile is used for a number of nervous system complaints including anxiety, premenstrual stress, menstrual cramps, menopausal depression, indigestion, and other digestive problems such as diarrhea, gastritis, colic, gas, stomach cramps, and loss of appetite. Its bittersweet taste lends it to being valuable in stimulating various gastric juices and improving digestion. The longer you let your chamomile flowers infuse in your teapot, twenty to thirty minutes, the more bitter they become and the more suitable the tea is for digestive problems.

Chamomile tea is safe and soothing for infants and children who are teething or who have colic or other stomach upsets. A homeopathic preparation made from chamomile, called chamomilla, is also readily available in health food stores and helps calm the body and spirit of an irritated and upset child and eases the uncomfortable symptoms associated with teething and colic.

A warm chamomile bath is a delightful gift at the end of a long day. You can add a few quarts of a strongly brewed chamomile tea to your bathwater or a few drops of the essential oil. A few drops of the essential oil placed in a pan of steaming (not boiling) water is a good way to breathe in the healing qualities of chamomile. Place your head over the steam and cover your head and the pan with a towel and breathe in the medicated steam for several minutes. The anti-inflammatory and antimicrobial properties of chamomile help heal inflamed mucous membrane linings of the lungs and sinuses and clears out excess mucus in the sinus cavities.

Picking chamomile flowers is one of my most favorite gardening activities. Mochi and I take a half-hour break from other more physically demanding garden tasks every few days in July to spend time with the chamomile. Mochi usually settles herself into the straw between the chamomile and mint beds while I hand-harvest a small basket full of chamomile flowers and then join her for a snooze.

CHICKWEED   (*Stellaria media*) *Caryophyllaceae*, Carnation
    Family
Other common names: Starwort, starweed, stitchwort, winterweed,
    white bird's eye
Parts used: Above-ground greens and tiny flowers

Various species of chickweed grow around our planet. The tiny white star-shaped flowers give away this plant in fields and gardens. Its Latin name, *Stellaria*, means little star. The leaves are smooth and oval shaped and the leaf stalks are hairy. Chickweed grows as an annual or biennial. The leaf stalks are 6–12 inches long and lay flat upon the soil.

Stellaria media is the most luscious of the chickweeds. Let this plant grow freely in a designated area in your garden and/or greenhouse, for its medicinal and edible uses are plentiful. It can be collected from early spring into late fall or winter (depending on where you live). Continuous harvesting of the greens prevents the plant from becoming stringy.

Its presence in the garden indicates nitrogen-rich soil. Chickweed came into our gardens in a load of cow manure. It now has a bed of its own that we continuously munch from and use for medicine.

Chickweed has a delicious, fresh taste and is high in minerals and vitamins. Eaten fresh in salads or taken as a tea or tincture, it soothes the digestive system, kidneys, bladder, urinary tract, lungs, and bowels. It is useful for people with internal ulcers to eat regularly.

Chickweed helps nutrients be absorbed into the body. It is a safe and nourishing herb for any age person who is weak, anemic, or recovering from a long-term illness or surgery to take every day over several weeks for gaining strength.

Chickweed is beneficial for women working to reduce and eliminate breast cysts, ovarian cysts, and uterine fibroids. Eat a few fresh handfuls chopped up in salad or added into soup as often as possible. If fresh chickweed is unavailable, take a tincture made from the fresh herb two to three times per day over several months along with any other healing methods you are utilizing. Continue using as a preventive measure when the growths disappear, or if you have the growths surgically removed.

A fresh chickweed poultice reduces swellings and inflammations from bruises, mosquito bites, and bee stings; relieves hot spots on an animal; and helps reduce hemorrhoids and heal skin ulcers and other inflamed or itchy skin conditions. A fresh poultice is also very effective for drawing out infections from abscesses, boils, cuts, and pus-filled wounds. A friend's nine-year-old dog's belly was recently covered with open, oozing, cancerous sores. Within three days of applying fresh chickweed poultices every few hours over the area, the infection drained, the odor lessened, and new pink cells formed. Soaking an inflamed or irritated area once or twice a day in a strong infusion of fresh chickweed is very soothing. A chickweed salve can ease itching of eczema or psoriasis and assist in the healing process of minor cuts and rashes.

A tea made from fresh chickweed leaves (in conjunction with herbs such as echinacea, goldenseal, and eyebright) and used as a wash relieves eye inflammations and helps heal eye infections, pink-eye, tired and sore eyes, and eyelids that may be crusted over. Chickweed is certainly an ally to the eyes and lungs of my friends who carve wood and build houses and wooden boats. Chickweed's demulcent properties are soothing to an irritated and inflamed respiratory tract and other inflamed organs.

Keep your eyes open for this tiny and extremely beneficial herb. Abundant Life Seed Foundation (listed in the Plant and Seed Resources list) sells chickweed seeds if you can't find plants from another garden to transplant into yours.

Chickweed Salad

Use whatever proportions of the following ingredients you feel inspired to use.

Large handful of freshly chopped chickweed

Grated carrots and beets

Alfalfa sprouts

Different colors and textures of lettuce

Chopped chives, parsley, lamb's quarters, and watercress

Add purple chive blossoms, borage flowers, nasturtium flowers, and Johnny-jump-up flowers when they are in the garden to garnish the top of the salad

Toasted sunflower seeds

A handful of toasted and crumbled dulse

Dressing

3 tablespoons of sesame tahini

1–2 tablespoons toasted sesame oil

¼ cup of yogurt, rice dream milk, or water

2–4 tablespoons of your favorite herb vinegar (I prefer using

a brown rice vinegar, apple cider vinegar, or umeboshi
plum vinegar)

1 tablespoon tamari sauce

1–2 medium cloves of freshly chopped garlic (or more if you
want)

LEMON BALM   (*Melissa officinalis*) *Labiatae*, Mint Family
Other common names: Melissa, balm, honeyplant
Parts used: Leaves and flowers. Most flavorful when used fresh in
   tea. Tincture fresh leaves and flowers. Dried leaves have a
   stronger flavor during the first six months after they are dried.

Lemon balm is commonly called melissa and is a fragrant
herb adored by honey bees. *Melissa* is the Greek word for honeybee.
In ancient European Goddess-worshipping cultures, bees were seen
"as a symbol of the feminine potency of nature, because they created this magical, good tasting substance and stored it in hexagonal
cells of geometric mystery."[3] Honey cakes shaped as female genitals
were often served at festivals honoring the Goddess.[4] If you are
interested in flower shapes, look at flowers in the *Labiatae* family
with a hand lens. You can see these flowers have lips, or labia, similar to the labia women have opening into our vaginas.

Priestesses of Aphrodite were called Melissa. In pre-Hellenic
mythology, Aphrodite was seen as a virgin, a woman one-in-herself,
independent, choosing who she would have sexual interactions
with. She was regarded as "a fertility Goddess, the primal mother of
all ongoing creation" and the maker of the morning dew.[5]

Melissa is native to southern Europe and has naturalized in
several places around the world including Asia, France, England,
and North and South America. The Romans were said to have introduced this plant to the British Isles where it became a plant of great
importance in the medicinal gardens of various monasteries.

The leaves are light green, deeply veined, and downy with
toothed margins, ovate to heart shaped, and two to three inches
long. They give off a fresh, lemony scent when gently rubbed

between your fingers. The stems branch out, are soft and hairy, and the pink and white flowers grow in whorls around the leaf axils and bloom from June to September. Lemon balm grows up to two feet high and is a tender perennial, especially in northern gardens. Mulching with straw or covering the plants with fir or pine boughs in the late fall helps them survive the winter. All fifty of my lemon balm plants, mulched thickly with straw, survived this past winter, which was very cold.

Melissa is easy to grow from seed. Start indoors, six weeks before transplanting into the garden, or sow directly into a well-prepared seed bed in the late fall or early spring. The plants self-sow freely if you let a few flower stalks go to seed instead of picking them. In some gardens, melissa can be found self-seeding everywhere and the seedlings make great gifts for friends. Large melissa plants can be divided with a spade in the springtime. Space seedlings or root divisions one foot apart.

Lemon balm grows in various soil conditions, but does best in a fertile, moist soil with a slightly acid to alkaline pH. I have observed over the years that plants grown in partial shade are greener and lusher than plants grown in full sun, which tend to be smaller and have yellower leaves.

Tea made from fresh lemon balm leaves and flowers is my favorite summer drink. You can easily cut the leaves and flower stalks with flower clippers or carefully pinch the leaves with your fingers. I often add a few fresh sprigs of sacred basil, sweet cicely leaves, and some borage and heartsease pansy flowers for a touch of fairy magic. When making tea from fresh leaves, I usually fill a glass cooking pot full of fresh lemon balm leaves, cover with water, and either let it sit in the sun for several hours or slowly warm it on the stove, not even to a simmer. I then remove the pan from the heat and steep, covered, for ten to thirty minutes.

To harvest and dry, carefully cut the flowering stalks before the flowers open. Lay the stalks and leaves on screens or tie in bunches and hang to dry. They will dry quickly, within a few days, if the weather is warm and sunny. Strip the leaves and flowers as soon as they are dry and store in glass jars with tightly fitting lids.

Melissa tea or tincture soothes and restores the nervous system, uplifts the spirit, and gladdens the heart. A cup of warm tea relieves anxiety and tension and eases uncomfortable menstrual cramps. Melissa in combination with lavender and St. Johnswort is a mild antidepression remedy. A warm cup of tea or a few drops of tincture helps bring on sleep, is calming to a child or adult after a nightmare, and can be given before bed to prevent further ones from occurring.

Warm melissa tea relieves spasms in the digestive tract and aids flatulent dyspepsia. It is useful for people who feel anxious and stressed to drink on a daily basis, to relieve tension and help prevent the digestive system from shutting down because of stress. Studies done in Germany show that the volatile oils in the spirits of melissa act upon the part of the brain that governs the autonomic nervous system and protects the cerebrum from excessive external stimuli. Lemon balm is an herb to seriously consider in the treatment of autonomic nervous disorders and for people on tranquilizers.[6]

Melissa helps reduce a mild fever and is safe for young children, the elderly, and pregnant and nursing mothers. Give ¼ to ½ cup of tea or 3–15 drops of tincture every half hour to hour, to lower a fever or calm an animal or person who is agitated from a sickness or emotional trauma.

A bath with a few drops of the pure essential oil of melissa, or a strong infusion of melissa tea added, is calming and comforting for anyone who feels overly anxious, stressed out, or exhausted. It is also soothing and calming for a pregnant woman or a woman in the early stages of labor, a woman experiencing menstrual cramps, or a woman experiencing heart palpitations, nervousness, migraine headaches, or insomnia with menopause. The soft glow of a candle, relaxing music, and a cup of warm lemon balm tea make nice bath companions.

NETTLES   (*Urtica dioica*) *Urticaceae*, Nettle Family
Other common names: Stinging nettle, wild spinach
Parts used: Spring leaves are used most often, though the seeds and
   root can also be utilized

Many people despise stinging nettles because the hairs on the stems and undersides of the leaves contain formic acid that stings some people. Many of us have probably had the experience or heard tales of people accidently running into a nettle patch. Bruised plantain or yellow dock leaves rubbed onto a sting will act as an antidote to the formic acid. Nettles can be an ally if you let yourself befriend this plant.

Stinging nettles grow wild in wet, rich soil in various places around the world. If you want to get a patch growing, the easiest way is to obtain a few cuttings and plant them in a shady area with plenty of compost or old manure and lots of room for them to spread. Plants growing in fertile soil can become over six feet high. A woman who lives near me planted nettles in her chicken yard twenty years ago and now has a large, luscious patch from which I am fortunate to be able to harvest. Keep your eyes open for nettles growing in your compost pile if you add cow manure to it. I now have two large beds of nettles growing in my garden that came in with a load of cow manure.

Nettle leaves are a dull green color, serrated, hairy, oval shaped, and grow opposite each other. Spring is the best time to gather the young leaves for eating, for tincturing, or for drying for tea. Take a pair of gloves and garden clippers. I cut the top three to four inches off the early spring plants. I am amused by the small, greenish yellow flowers that hang down from the stems in early summer. The female and male flowers grow on separate plants or branches. The seeds can be collected in early fall when they turn brown.

By the time spring arrives in Maine, I am desperate for fresh greens and spring-picked nettles steamed for a few minutes and eaten with brown rice, toasted ground sesame seeds, and flax-seed oil is a delicious treat that I eat several times a week. The formic acid wilts when the leaves are steamed or cooked in soups or casseroles and will not sting you. One April I spent two weeks hiking in the mountains of North Carolina and Tennessee and the young spring nettles were growing everywhere. We ate steamed nettles every night and were so happy to have this fresh tasty green to supplement our dinners. I did not tire of eating them, and every spring I eagerly await steamed nettle greens. They are a wonderful spring tonic and detoxifying remedy.

Another delicious way to eat nettles is to layer them instead of spinach into a spanakopita. Herbalist Rosemary Gladstar turned me on to nettle spanakopita. Her recipe is written in one of the pamphlets she publishes called *Rosemary's Wild Food Recipes.* They are available for $4.50 through the mail (SAGE, P.O. Box 420, East Barre, VT 05649).

To dry the leaves, pick them in the spring before the flowers form and before the plants are three feet high. Carefully lay them onto nylon screens. Once dry, the hairs may feel prickly if you handle the leaves with your bare hands, but the formic acid is gone. Store the leaves in glass jars in a dark place.

Nettle leaves are high in iron and safe to drink as a daily tea or several times a week, especially good for women who are anemic. A nettle tea or tincture, taken internally over several weeks, strengthens the kidneys and adrenal glands, nourishes the liver and blood, and improves the elasticity of the veins. Anyone with hemorrhoids or varicose veins will benefit from drinking 1–3 cups of nettle tea daily for several weeks or months. Nettle also strengthens the outer membrane (also called plasma membrane) of cells, making them less vulnerable to inflammation and allergic reactions.

Nettle leaves are safe for pregnant and nursing women. Daily use of nettle-leaf tea or fresh tincture in combination with yellow dock root tincture or tea raises the body's iron level significantly. Nettle tea, alone, or in combination with other herbs such as red raspberry leaves, borage leaves, and fennel seed, is a nourishing postpartum tea for rebuilding strength and adding nutrients to breast milk. Nettles and yellow dock replenish iron in women who have lost large amounts of blood during childbirth, surgery, or heavy menstrual flow. Take two to four times per day for several weeks or months.

Nettles are a friend to women experiencing menopause. Warm nettle and sage-leaf tea helps reduce night sweats, and nettles in combination with other herbs such as oatstraw, red raspberry leaves, borage leaves, and Siberian ginseng, support the body through this changing time by increasing low energy levels and helping overcome fatigue.

Nettle is an excellent herb to add into a formula for eczema and various skin eruptions, including hot spots on animals. Take it internally and use it as a wash externally.

Warm nettle tea helps the body to release excess mucus from the lungs and colon. Fresh nettle tea or tincture is also beneficial for people with hay fever, asthma, and frequent nosebleeds. Its astringent properties lessen nosebleeds, uterine hemorrhages, and bleeding from cuts.

Nettle tea taken cool helps reduce inflammatory conditions of the bladder and kidneys. I have also seen some people and animals with arthritis or rheumatism have their symptoms subside with daily use of nettle tea or tincture.

A nettle tea rinse stimulates hair growth for people and animals. Let the leaves steep in cool water for eight hours, strain, and use the tea once or twice a week to rinse your hair. Nettle leaves, sage, rosemary, chamomile, and lavender flowers can be added to apple cider vinegar and left soaking for one month. Strain, and use 1 tablespoon of the vinegar to 1 cup of water as a hair rinse.

Powdered nettle leaves combined with powdered alfalfa, rosemary, and kelp are an excellent dietary supplement for dogs, cats, horses, goats, llamas, chickens, cows, and sheep. The skin, hair, and bones of any animal look and feel healthier with daily use of these nourishing herbs added to their food. I have given this combination to my dog and to dozens of other animals for several years. The feedback people give regarding the improvement in their animal's health and vitality is astounding.

I saw a variety of nettles growing in many mountainous villages in eastern Nepal on my most recent visit, in 1992. The whole plant is harvested in September, then the bark from the main stalk is stripped, cooked in wood ash water, pounded in running water, spun into a fiber, and woven into a durable, nonitchy cloth. Nettle was widely used for making cloth in many places throughout Europe until the beginning of the twentieth century.

The most effective way I know of extracting the various minerals nettle contains is by placing the dried or fresh leaves in a glass pot of cool water and letting it sit overnight. The tea water will be brownish in the morning. Sometimes I drink this tea cool, or I warm it up slowly and then let it steep for five to fifteen minutes.

OATS (*Avena sativa, fatua*, and other species) *Graminacaceae*, Grain Family
Other common names: Wild oats, avena
Parts used: Fresh green milky seeds, straw, and grain

Oats grow wild in some places in the United States and other countries and are also widely cultivated around the world. Oats came into our gardens with cow manure and volunteered to grow in a specific bed, much to my delight. I enjoy watching the green seeds swell in early summer and later, as they ripen, listening to them whisper and rattle as they sway in the wind.

The fresh, green seeds are harvested when they are plump and in the milky stage. Squeeze some seeds in your fingers, and if white milk oozes out they are ready to pick. Tincture them immediately after harvesting. The ripened seeds and straw are harvested in late summer for grain and tea. The stalks are cut, tied, and left to dry upright and out of the weather. Once dry, the seed is threshed out and the straw broken up and stored for tea.

Oat

Oats are one of my favorite herbs for feeding and nourishing the nervous system. Daily use of oats slowly increases overall strength, energy, and calmness, states of being that many people living and working in stressful situations need help in creating. As a nerve tonic, oatstraw tea and fresh tincture support the nervous system of a person who is exhausted, tense, anxious, or depressed. Oats are valuable for people whose nervous systems have been overstimulated by abuse of drugs, alcohol, fast-paced lifestyles, or poor quality foods; for people recovering from illnesses, including nervous breakdowns; and for elderly people. They are also a remedy I encourage people who experience nervous headaches, heart palpitations, nerve tremors, nervous dyspepsia, mental exhaustion, and epileptic seizures to incorporate into their health plans.

Oat tincture and oatstraw tea are safe for pregnant and nursing women and beneficial because of their nutritive and tonic properties. The high silica content found in oats assists in the development of strong bones, teeth, hair, and nails. Also, eating plenty of cooked and organic steel-cut or rolled oats on a regular basis benefits the whole nervous system, whether you are pregnant or not.

Oats are a nourishing herb for women to take several times a week throughout their years of menstruating, during pregnancy, through menopause, and beyond. A strong infusion made by steeping 4–8 ounces of dried oatstraw in 2 quarts of steaming hot water, covered, for thirty minutes, strained and added to a bath is very soothing and restorative. A poultice made from cooked rolled oats helps to relieve itchy skin, and powdered oats mixed with white clay, ground almonds, and water makes a wonderful paste for cleansing the face. After washing off the paste I sometimes smother my face with honey and leave it on for fifteen minutes. This brings blood to the surface and softens the skin.

RED CLOVER BLOSSOMS   (*Trifolium pratense*) *Leguminosaea*,
   Pea Family
Other common names: Purple clover, meadow trefoil
Part used: Blossom

Red clover is commonly found growing in hay fields and can be planted on the edge of gardens. It blooms early to mid June in Maine and again in August and September in fields that were mowed during the summer. Many of you may remember eating the pinkish red blossoms when you were children. They are a nutritious and beautiful addition to any salad.

Red clover is a member of the legume family and grows as a biennial. The leaves are oval shaped and divided into three finely toothed leaflets. The plant sends down a strong tap root that has nitrogen-fixing nodules on it. Wherever clovers grow, the nitrogen content in the soil increases.

The field next to our gardens is covered with red clover blossoms and various other wildflowers. I enjoy watching this hillside come into bloom and go to seed throughout the summer. The yellow dandelion flowers are the first to come, followed by red clover, blue vetch, white yarrow, yellow rattle, pink meadowsweet, and orange wood lilies. One morning my neighbor's eight-year-old daughter came out to see which flowers I was gathering. I explained to her some of their medicinal uses. She exclaimed that if she was ever sick it should be at her father's house as his field contained all the medicine she might need.

To make red clover tea, soak the flowers in cool water overnight to extract the minerals. If you want to drink warm tea, then slowly heat the tea and steep, covered, for ten to fifteen minutes. Red clover helps clear the blood of waste products during or after a sickness or during a seasonal change. Drink 2–5 cups a day when coming down with a cold, fever, or flu. Red clover's antispasmodic and expectorant properties make it effective for treating coughs, bronchitis, and whooping cough. It is safe for children, pregnant and nursing women, and elderly people, and it's a good herb to combine with others because it adds a mild, sweet taste to tea.

Red clover is an excellent addition to a tea formula for skin problems such as acne, skin ulcers, eczema, and psoriasis. A strong infusion of red clover blossoms—strong meaning the blossoms are infused in cool water for eight hours—is beneficial to use as a rinse on open sores and inflamed skin, burns, skin ulcers, and hot spots on animals. Red clover can be made into a poultice, or fomentation, and is a wonderful herb to add to an all-purpose herb salve for healing mild cuts and skin rashes.

Recent studies show that red clover blossoms contain the chemical genistiene, also found in soy beans, which inhibits the spread of cancer. Red clover tea is a safe and nourishing herb to drink several times a week over several months. You can drink it alone or in combination with other herbs.

Keep your eyes open for the first signs of red clover in the summer. Give yourself a few sunny mornings to enjoy gathering some baskets full of flowers to dry and store for the winter. Red clover harvesting can be a nice meditative ritual to do alone or with a friend. If you have children, or are with children who are eager to help you pick, then an adventure may be in store for you.

Pick the blossoms that are fresh, vibrant, and colorful. Avoid blossoms that have begun to turn brown. Brown, tasteless red clover is usually what you will find commercially. Compare the flavor and feel of wild-harvested red clover to commercial grade. The vitality and sweetness of the clover you gather yourself will delight your taste buds. As soon as you come in from picking, spread the flowers out on nylon screens to dry. They dry fairly quickly, often within a few days, if the weather is sunny and warm. Check them each day and store in a glass jar with a good fitting lid once you are sure they are dry. Overdrying will cause the flowers to fall apart and their strength and vitality to be less.

If you want, take time to look closely at a fresh red clover blossom under a hand lens. Each flowerlet looks like tiny wings that resemble the flowery opening of a woman's vagina. Flowers have a wonderful way of mirroring back to us the beauty of our own bodies and reminding us of our inherent strength and goodness.

RED RASPBERRY LEAVES   (*Rubus idaeus*) *Rosaceae*, Rose Family
Parts used: Leaves from first-year canes that are not flowering; enjoy
   the delectable fruits from the second-year canes

Red raspberry grows wild in the more northern areas of the United States and Canada. You will often find thickets growing in fields, hedgerows, and by old foundations. Many of the islands off the Maine coast are covered with wild raspberries—a special treat for kayakers to find in August.

The upright canes grow from underground suckers and stolons and range from three to six feet in height. The canes are usually a bit prickly to touch. The green leaves are toothed, have three to five leaflets, and are a distinctly gray or whitish color on their underside. The small white flowers grow in clusters and bloom in Maine in June. The red fruit appears in August.

Leaves gathered from wild, uncultivated plants are strongest. If you only have access to organically cultivated red raspberries, then do gather what you find. Collect leaves from the first-year canes, plants that are not yet producing flowers and berries. They cut easily with clippers and can be harvested throughout the summer on sunny mornings. Lay them out on screens immediately after harvesting. They dry quickly when the weather is sunny and hot. Check them daily so they will not overdry. Picking raspberry leaves is a special event to share with other women since this plant offers so many gifts to women. Be sure to gather enough to last you through the winter and to share with your women friends. A gallon of dried leaves goes quickly when raspberry tea is taken daily.

Red raspberry leaves are an excellent uterine tonic, serving to strengthen and tone the muscles of the uterus. They contain a substance called fragrine. Fragrine has a special affinity for the muscles of the pelvic area and the uterus, which is why red raspberry is so highly regarded for its use during pregnancy, labor, and immediately after birth. It is an excellent uterine tonic for all women, regardless of whether they are pregnant.

Our womb area is the center of our divine understanding. It is the place in our bodies from which we deeply feel and intuit things. Keeping our hormonal system strong and balanced ensures balance of our whole body. One to three cups of raspberry tea taken daily, or several times during the week, will tone the uterus and restore strength to the hormonal system. Regular use of raspberry leaves eases premenstrual discomforts, and helps reduce, and in some cases eliminate, menstrual cramps after extended use. Daily use supports hormonal changes during pregnancy and after giving birth, after a miscarriage or abortion, throughout menopause, after a hysterectomy or any surgery in the pelvic area, when coming off the pill or other hormone drugs and steroids, and when recovering from alcohol or drug abuse.

I include raspberry leaf in tea formulas for women who are healing from any form of sexual abuse, rape, and when incest memories are resurfacing. Many women begin to remember early childhood traumas later in life when circumstances in their lives trigger a memory and a door reopens. Refer to the section on healing from sexual abuse in chapter 8 for more herbal information.

Raspberry leaf tea in combination with other herbs supports a woman who is grieving the loss of a loved one who is connected energetically to her womb, such as her mother, grandmother, lover, or child. Raspberry tea supports losses that are recent or old. The cells in our bodies remember all our experiences.

Raspberry leaves mix well with a variety of herbs, including nettle, red clover, alfalfa, chamomile, linden flowers, oatstraw, calendula, hawthorn flowers, lemon balm, and whatever else you like. Drink raspberry leaf tea warm or cool. Experiment with steeping the leaves for different lengths of time to see what you like. When steeped for twenty to thirty minutes raspberry tea tastes bitter to some women. Better to let your tea steep less than to not drink its nourishing gifts. Freezing raspberry tea with a few teaspoons of honey into ice cubes is an easy way to offer a woman in labor raspberry tea and something refreshing to chew on.

4

Sea Vegetables

Call us not weeds; we are flowers of the Sea.

—UNKNOWN

SEAWEED NICHES

Of the intertidal zone on a rocky Maine coast promontory

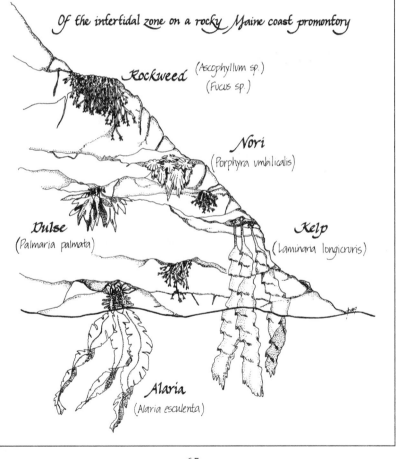

Rockweed (Ascophyllum sp.)
(Fucus sp.)

Nori (Porphyra umbilicalis)

Dulse (Palmaria palmata)

Kelp (Laminaria longicruris)

Alaria (Alaria esculenta)

Sea vegetables are eaten on a regular basis by many coastal people around the world and are extremely nourishing to the body because of their high vitamin, mineral, and trace element content. They contain fifty-six mineral and trace elements needed by the body for optimum health, along with other valuable nutrients that counteract the adverse effects of radiation, heavy metals, and other environmental pollutants.[1]

Studies done at McGill University in Montreal show that sodium alginate, present in sea vegetables belonging to the kelp family (*Phaephyceae*), protects the body from radioactive and environmental contaminants, including strontium 90.[2] (Strontium 90 is a radionuclide released by atomic explosions that can cause serious health problems.) Some of the sea vegetables found in the kelp family are *Alaria esculenta*, similar to the Japanese wakame, *Laminaria longicruris*, known as kombu or kelp or fucus, and *Ascophyllum species*, commonly called rockweed or bladderwrack.

Sea vegetables are an important addition to our daily diets because of the ever-increasing amounts of radioactive waste and chemical poisons present in our environment. Strontium 90 is found in most people's bones today. Statistics show that the adverse effects of its presence in our bones increases with time and are responsible for the higher incidences of the following conditions and diseases: anemia, bone cancer, leukemia, Hodgkin's disease, and the decreased production of red and white blood cells.[3]

Radioactive strontium and other pollutants are in our food chain because of the modern world's production of toxic chemicals and its horrendous, unsafe dumping practices. When contaminated water or food is ingested, the poisons enter the bloodstream via the small intestine and are deposited in the bones. The sodium alginate in kelps binds with the radioactive strontium and other metal pollutants—lead, barium, cadmium, excess iron—and changes them into an insoluble gel-like salt. This salt is then eliminated from the body through the feces. The red sea vegetables, such as dulse

(*Palmaria palmata*), have proven to be the most effective at binding with plutonium, and the green algaes such as sea lettuce are most effective at binding with cesium. Be sure to increase intake of sea vegetables before, during, and after any exposure to X-rays, radiation, or chemotherapy.

Research shows that sodium alginate is nontoxic and that eating the kelps on a daily basis is the most effective way to protect the body from radioactive poisoning and environmental pollutants. The body's digestive, endocrine, cardiovascular, immune, and nervous systems also benefit from a daily intake of seaweeds.

Substances such as steroids, birth control pills, antibiotics, and highly processed foods destroy the villi in the small intestines. Different kinds of stresses—emotional, mental, or physical—cause the villi in the small intestines to atrophy. Car exhaust, smoke, gaseous fumes, wood dust, and other forms of air pollution harm the villi in the lungs.

Daily intake of the kelps helps heal colitis, an ulcerated colon, and gastric and duodenal ulcers; balances acid-alkaline levels in the gastrointestinal tract; improves the assimilation of nutrients into the bloodstream, thus improving overall health; and soothes irritated lung tissues.[4]

The mineral and vitamin content of sea vegetables improves the health of the cardiovascular and nervous systems by nourishing the heart muscle, improving the tissue integrity of blood vessels and veins, reducing varicosities, strengthening circulation, evening out blood pressure, feeding the various nerve pathways, improving mental alertness and memory, and lessening the effects of mental stress, thus allowing one to think more clearly.

Seaweeds contain natural iodine, which feeds the thyroid gland, prevents the assimilation of radioactive iodine by the thyroid gland, and ensures that the nervous system is functioning well. Deficient levels of iodine in the diet affect the thyroid's ability to direct the body's metabolic processes. This causes the immune system to become weakened and sets the body up for dis-ease.[5]

Seaweeds offer specific nourishment and healing for women. They come from the sea, whose ebbing and flowing rhythms and deep dark waters are so much like our wombs, our menstrual cycles, and our dreamtime. The depths of the ocean are rich in life and mysterious in a way similar to the depths of our bodies and psyches. Spend time walking and sitting by the sea if you live near-by. Go for a swim if the water is warm enough, or run barefoot along the water's edge. Let your whole being be filled with the sounds of the waves, seabirds, and, if you are lucky, with the songs of the seals and whales.

The daily eating of seaweeds restores and increases our vitali-ty and energy by remineralizing our bodies. Kelps help prevent, reduce, and eliminate fibrocystic breast tissue, ovarian cysts, uterine fibroids, menstrual cramps, and hot flashes.[6] The following is excerpted from an article in the journal *Medical Hypotheses*.

> A review of the biological properties of seaweed is present-ed and the role of seaweed as a breast cancer anticarcinogen is suggested. Proposed mechanisms of action are: reduction of plas-ma cholesterol, binding of biliary steroids, inhibition of carcino-genic fecal flora, binding of pollutants, stimulation of the immune system, and the protective effects of beta-sitosterols.[7]

The high mineral content present in all seaweeds helps pre-vent osteoporosis and promotes fertility. Wakame is considered by macrobiotics to be particularly supportive for women's reproduc-tive organs and regulating the menstrual cycle. Linnette Erhart from Maine Coast Sea Vegetables wrote to me,

> Before my first successful pregnancy, I ate lots of alaria (like wakame), which grows at the lowest tide zone, an area of intense wave action. Alaria has tremendous tenacity in a watery environ-ment. I am convinced that this helped bring about a successful embryonic attachment. The placenta and cord bear uncanny resemblance to the holdfast (part of the alaria which is like the placenta that connects the stipe and frond to the rocks) and stipe (cord that connects the leafy frond and holdfast).

Alaria, arame, wakame, hiziki, dulse, kelp, nori, and agar-agar are some of the most commonly available sea vegetables on the market in the United States, though over seventy-five species are eaten around the world. Soaking the seaweed before cooking and discarding the soaking water dramatically decreases the sodium content to levels that are safe even for people with heart problems.[8] One-half to one ounce of cooked seaweed is a good amount to eat on a daily basis (more is recommended for therapeutic situations). Remember to also mix ¼–2 teaspoons of granulated kelp into your pet's food every day.

If you do not eat seaweeds, try 5–10 tablets of kelp daily, or use a high quality kelp extract. Or look for secondary sea vegetable products for healthy snacks, such as corn chips with dulse, kelp pickles, crackers, sea vegetable seasonings, and kelp candy. Many of these products are made by Maine Coast Sea Vegetables and are delicious. Look for them in health food stores, or you can mail order from them directly (their address is listed in the resource list).

The Division of Biomedical and Environmental Research of the Atomic Energy Commission recommends that if someone is directly exposed to radiation she increase the daily dosage of sodium alginate to 2 full tablespoons, four times per day, to insure that the gastrointestinal tract has a sufficient and continuous supply of sodium alginate.

I am fortunate to live near the sea. Besides being able to enjoy the smell of the salt air, the full moon rising over the water, and the magical images the fog creates in my gardens, I collect truckloads of rockweed each spring and fall, with the help of friends, for mulching Avena's gardens and for layering into the compost pile. The rockweeds add important minerals to the soil and break down easily.

It is important to note that when collecting or purchasing seaweeds for food or your garden they should be harvested from relatively pollution-free areas—away from industrial harbors and major shipping channels. Shep Erhart, of Maine Coast Sea Vegetables, now has his products tested for contaminants and has been working on organic certification standards for sea vegetables. Carefully read the packaging of sea vegetable products to determine if the producer is concerned about pollution and processing. Shep says the careful ways the harvester handles and processes the sea vegetables are also crucial to the overall quality of the plants, just the same as when gathering fresh herbs for drying or tincturing.

Miso-Seaweed Soup

Place 1–2, 6-inch strips of kelp in a pot with 1½ cups water and bring to a boil. Add 1–3 teaspoons of herbs, such as basil or thyme, cover, and simmer for twenty minutes. Remove the kelp, cut into ½-inch squares, and return to the pot. Thinly slice any of the following vegetables into small pieces: onion, carrot, beet, parsnip, lovage or celery stalk, or burdock root and simmer for ten minutes. Then add in a few leaves of kale, dandelion, yellow dock, or nettles and simmer until everything is tender. I like to add in chopped garlic at the end of cooking and add a teaspoon of brown rice miso to each individual bowl of soup and garnish with toasted dulse, parsley, and/or chickweed.

Buttercup Stew With Wakame and Dulse

Boil 4–6 cups of water. Cut 6–12 inches of wakame into small pieces and place into soup pot with 2–3 teaspoons of sweet marjoram and simmer for five to ten minutes. Then add in 3–4 cups of buttercup squares, 3 cups of Jerusalem artichokes, 2–3 potatoes (if you eat potatoes), and 1–2 leeks, thinly sliced. Simmer for ten to fifteen minutes; add in a chopped lovage or celery stalk and 2 cups of cooked adzuki beans. Simmer another fifteen minutes, or longer if needed. Add freshly chopped garlic. Dissolve 2 tablespoons of kuzu into ¼ cup of cool water and stir into the stew until it thickens. Add barley or brown rice miso to taste and crumble whatever amount of lightly toasted dulse you like on top along with chopped parsley.

5

Nourishing Our Roots

The truth is
I have mud on my hands
from digging roots
The truth is
I brought them to you
It is the truth
I worked to get them
and complained
while digging them up
The truth is
once I got back here
and saw your face
it didn't matter,
that work

—SWAMPY CREE INDIAN

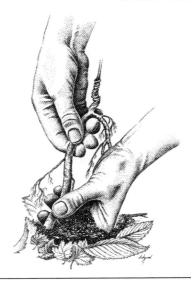

71

THE LIVER

The liver is the largest organ in the body and carries out many diverse jobs. It manufactures bile, which breaks down fats; stores the fat-soluble vitamins such as A, D, E, K, and other vitamins and minerals; metabolizes carbohydrates, fats, and proteins; filters the bloodstream of waste products normally produced in the body; detoxifies fat soluble drugs, barbiturates, and environmental toxins; destroys old, worn-out red blood cells; helps maintain electrolyte and water balance; and provides a place for extra blood to be stored and quickly released if needed. Certain cells in the liver can also regenerate themselves after becoming diseased or being injured as long as the disease has not progressed past a certain point.

For women, the health of the liver is significant because it breaks down and eliminates excess levels of hormones such as estrogen, the corticosteroids, and other steroids. An overstressed and congested liver is less able to deal with peak levels of sex hormones associated with premenstrual stress, especially from ovulation through to the onset of menses. This can lead to a wide range of discomforts such as water retention, swollen breasts, cramping, mood swings, depression, fatigue, sluggish digestion, diarrhea, constipation, migraine headaches, and feelings of disharmony, anger, and frustration.

When the liver is not properly functioning, the whole body is affected. The skin, kidneys, heart, glandular, immune, or digestive system may show signs of weakness or imbalance. If you experience chronic problems in any of these areas, seek qualified medical help from an experienced holistic practitioner.

Fortunately, there are many safe and effective herbs that help to decongest and strengthen the liver. The liver's health will also greatly increase by reducing the intake of fat, drugs, alcohol, caffeine, nicotine, sugar, and highly processed foods.

The roots of plants in particular can be deeply cleansing and nourishing to the liver and improve overall digestion. Root teas and tinctures are often used for people with long-term health imbalances since roots can work on a deep level, helping a person to understand and change the underlying root cause of their illness. The following are some of my favorite herbs for supporting the liver and improving digestion. Various roots also support the body during seasonal changes and are listed in a chart at the end of this chapter called Living in Harmony With the Seasons.

LIVER HERBS

BLESSED THISTLE   (*Cnicus benedictus*)
   Compositae, Daisy Family
Other common names: Holy thistle, lady's
   thistle
Parts used: Leaves and flowers and
   root

   Blessed thistle is native to the Mediterranean area, has naturalized itself in central and southeastern Europe, and is cultivated in medicinal gardens in various parts of the world. Being a thistle, it is easy to start from seed and grows as an annual in my Maine gardens. Each fall I collect the seeds for starting seedlings indoors the following March. A botanist friend of mine once told me that blessed thistle was grown in monastic gardens during the time of the European witch-hunts.

Blessed Thistle

How wonderful, I thought, that the Catholic nuns and monks were making sure some of the healing herbs were kept alive despite the Catholic church's role in killing women herbalists.
   My favorite time to sit with these plants is at dawn when they are covered with dew and the sun's first rays shine through the flowers, illuminating them. The green leaves are prickly and lance shaped and the upper leaves enfold the yellowish green flowers that begin flowering midsummer. This sprawling plant grows one to two feet high and its branching stems are reddish and downy.

Blessed thistle grows well in sunny, well-drained garden spots and in soil that has some compost mixed in.

We harvest the leaves and flowers for drying and tincturing in midsummer and then again in early fall before the killing frost. The leaves are extremely bitter tasting and my hands and mouth taste bitter for one to two days after harvesting. When collecting seeds, keep a close watch on how the seeds are maturing. I check various seed heads regularly to be sure they have ripened fully before harvesting them. In hotter climates the plants reseed themselves freely.

Blessed thistle is an ally for women. It is an herb I use in combination with the roots of a Chinese herb called bupleurum for women who are feeling overly angry or frustrated, or who have a history of anorexia or poor digestion. Blessed thistle and dandelion root support a regular and healthy menstrual flow by toning the liver and balancing menstrual and menopausal discomforts that are the result of a congested liver. Blessed thistle is nourishing to mother's milk and mixes well with fennel or anise seed, nettles, raspberry, borage, and mints.

Blessed thistle is an excellent herb for aiding weakened digestion and toning the liver and spleen. It helps when digestion feels slowed down and painful and the abdomen is distended. Its bitter properties stimulate bile flow and hydrochloric acid production, thereby improving assimilation of nutrients and increasing overall health. Blessed thistle is particularly important for menopausal women, who often have low hydrochloric acid levels. Christopher Hobbs suggests in his book, *Foundations of Health: The Liver and Digestive Herbal*, to take blessed thistle in cycles, ten days on, three days off, ten days on, etc.

BURDOCK   (*Arctium lappa*) *Compositae*, Daisy Family
Other common names: Clotbur, gobo, fox's clote, beggar's buttons,
   wooly dock
Parts used: First-year roots, seeds, and leaves

Burdock originated in Europe and is now widespread throughout the world. It is a biennial and reseeds itself prolifically, especially in gardens, ditches, along roadsides, and near barns. The leaves are grayish green and rough textured. The first year's growth

NOURISHING OUR ROOTS / 75

produces large basal leaves in a rosette shape. These leaves can grow up to one and a half foot long and have a grayish fuzz on the underside.

A first-year plant does not have a flower stalk. Roots are dug for food and medicine in the spring and fall of the first year. The taproot is long, fleshy, slightly aromatic, and brown on the outside and white inside. Burdock can be difficult to dig because of its long taproot and because it often grows wild in hard-packed soil. Loosen the soil around the leaves and root with a shovel before attempting to pull. After a few times of pulling and the root snapping off, you'll get the hang of it. If you are gathering wild burdock, be sure to check with someone to make certain the land has not been sprayed or been used as a dumping ground, and to ask permission. After digging roots, I encourage people to spread the soil around and leave the area looking like you had not been there.

A thick, three- to five-foot stalk grows from the center the second year, and the leaves become smaller as they ascend upward, ending with small, purple, thistlelike flowers. As the flowers fade, the bristles stiffen, become stickier, and the burrs form. A six-foot-high burdock with many branching arms grew in front of the steps to our house one summer. I called her the guardian of the house. I talked to her frequently, thanking her for protecting us and letting her know that when the sticky burrs formed we would need to respectfully saw her flowerstalk off so the many hummingbirds who flew nearby would not get caught and die as I have seen happen before.

Burdock grows everywhere. We are blessed by the abundance of this wild weed, though many people who do not know of burdock's healing virtues disagree. Burdock is easy to cultivate in raised beds, which makes digging roots much easier. The Japanese call the root *gobo* and cook with it frequently. We store the roots in our root cellar for putting in winter soups and vegetable stir-fries. I have used the fresh leaves of first-year plants and roots as a wash for animals whose skin is dry, irritated, and flaky. A leaf infusion is also great as a hair rinse for humans with dandruff.

Burdock root eaten, or used as a tea or tincture, is nourishing for the liver and kidneys and promotes digestion and appetite through the bitter stimulation of digestive juices and the secretion of bile. It helps eliminate ingested chemicals and the waste materials normally produced by the body. Burdock root is used in anti-cancer remedies because it helps to inactivate cancer-causing agents. Burdock-root tea is also beneficial for healing cystitis, an inflammation of the bladder.[1]

I often drink 3–4 cups of burdock tea when I feel myself coming down with a cold or flu as a way to support my body's eliminative channels. Burdock root in combination with dandelion roots, yellow dock roots, and nettle is one of my favorite spring tonics. You can benefit from its tonic effects by drinking 1–3 cups per day or taking the tincture one to three times per day for six weeks in the spring.

Burdock root and seeds are a good remedy to take internally, either in tincture or tea form, for any skin affliction like acne, eczema, psoriasis, herpes sores, boils, or sebaceous eruptions. I have seen burdock root tincture, taken internally, three to four times a day for seven to ten days, and plantain oil applied topically, clear up ringworm within a week. For persistent ringworm apply a few drops of undiluted ti tree oil directly on the patches.

Burdock seeds, taken internally as tea or tincture, are more specific for healing scaly skin problems than the root. If you want to collect seeds, pick them in the fall after the purple color has faded. Separate the seeds from the chaff by winnowing them, crushing them with a rolling pin, or putting them in a blender.

Note: Michael Moore writes in *Medicinal Plants of the Mountain West* that the ingestion of burdock seeds should be avoided by pregnant women until the last trimester, as they could possibly cause some spotting.

DANDELION   (*Taraxacum officinale*)   *Compositae*, Daisy Family
Other common names: Lion's tooth, bitterwort, piss-in-bed
Parts used: Roots, leaves, and flowers

Dandelion roots can be unearthed in the spring or fall and used fresh or dried in teas and soups and, preferably, used fresh when making tincture. They are considered by many herbalists to be more of a liver tonic when dug in the late winter or spring than when dug in the fall. The leaves can be eaten in salads, steamed, or

cooked in soups as far into the summer
as one wants. The flowers make a colorful addition to salads. They are
delicious as a tempura in a batter of flour, milk, and eggs for
a special spring treat (recipe
listed below).

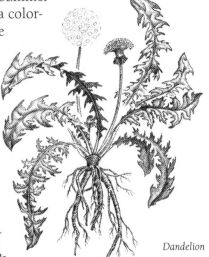

There is nothing more
delightful for me in spring
than a hillside ablaze with yellow dandelion flowers. Every
spring I marvel at individual
dandelion flowers in my garden, each flower a perfect mandala, alive with buzzing insects of
all kinds. Dandelion flowers con-

Dandelion

tinue to teach me to take nothing for granted. Though I have collected hundreds of plants, they remind me to not tire of the constant and unique beauty of each plant and every moment.

Different dandelion species are found around the world. The
leaf of the plant varies; some are deeply toothed and others just
slightly cut. A hollow, red-colored stem grows from the center of a
rosette of leaves, which grows flat on the ground. The bright yellow
flower heads are one to two inches in diameter. A milky juice comes
out of the stems when they are broken. The taproot is brown on the
outside and white inside.

Dandelion roots are easy to dig with a spade. Keep your eyes
open in the springtime for the old-timers out collecting dandelion
greens. Usually they are people in their fifties or older who carry on
their family's tradition of eating the spring greens of dandelion.

I feel strongly that the chemical weed killers some people use
to wipe out dandelions in their lawns should be banned. People
would be healthier all around if they ate dandelion greens and
drank root tea instead of jeopardizing their liver's health, and the
health of soil, water, animals, and insects with insecticides and pesticides. In 1990, over thirty million pounds of insecticides were
applied to residential gardens and lawns in the United States.[2] This
money could be funneled instead into health care, domestic vio-

lence programs, child care facilities and schools, organic farming pilot programs . . . etc.

Dandelion root is the first herb I call upon for women to use to decongest the liver and keep it from becoming overburdened by excess amounts of hormones. I recommend women drinking dandelion root tea, or taking the tincture, one to three times daily, five days a week, for four to six weeks in the spring and fall, and using it three to four times per week other times of the year as a nourishing and liver tonic herb. When working with a chronic menstrual problem, use two to three times a day, five days a week for many months. Many women have told me that consistent use of dandelion root over one to six months cleared up many menstrual difficulties they had like cramping, water retention, and pelvic congestion, and helped balance their feelings of extreme frustration or anger.

Dandelion root tea or tincture is valuable for women going through menopause to take on a regular, long-term basis for helping regulate hormonal changes. It is also safe and effective for protecting the liver for women who are taking estrogen replacement or other hormonal drugs. The liver works extra hard to digest foreign chemicals and hormones. Use dandelion one to three times a day, four to five days a week for as long as you are on a hormonal replacement therapy.

Dandelion root is safe for pregnant and nursing women to take a few times a week to assist the liver in processing the hormonal changes that occur during pregnancy and after giving birth. If you are planning to become pregnant, begin taking dandelion-root tea or tincture one to two times a day, for one to three months before you begin trying to conceive.

The roots ease inflammation of the liver and gallbladder, improve bile disorders and constipation, and help to prevent the formation of gallstones and gravel. Dandelion roots are helpful to use in formulas for clearing up jaundice, hepatitis, and when treating muscular rheumatism.

Dandelion leaves are an excellent diuretic. They contain potassium, which is leached from the body by chemical diuretics. Whenever water retention is a problem, call upon dandelion leaves to help. You can eat them, dry the spring leaves for tea, or make a fresh tincture from spring leaves.

Dandelion root offers liver support for people who are recovering from drug or alcohol abuse, overextended use of antibiotics, and eating disorders. People healing from a long-term liver problem will benefit from taking dandelion root tea or tincture one to two times per day, three to four times a week, for several months.

Spring and fall are the most beneficial times of the year to strengthen and tone the liver. The liver works hard to digest the fattier foods that people living in northern climates often eat during the winter. The liver appreciates extra nourishment when spring comes so that it can continue to do its numerous jobs. As spring approaches, we begin to eat different foods, the blood begins to thin, and the body's temperature changes—spring cleaning. The fall finds the body making similar adjustments in preparation for winter, and the stronger the liver is the easier these transitions occur.

Roots dry well on nylon screens hung above a wood stove, in a warm attic out of the direct sunlight, or in a gas oven with a pilot flame. Be sure to put a big sign that says HERBS DRYING IN OVEN so you won't turn on the oven and destroy the roots. The ideal temperature for drying roots and herbs is 85–100°F. Above 100°F, the essential oils and other chemical constituents begin to be destroyed.

Digging roots is a special way to get your hands into the soil and to connect with the earth's wisdom. Dandelion is a gift to us because she grows abundantly and is easily accessible.

Dandelion Flower Tempura

Get on your rubber boots and with basket in hand go out to your garden or a nearby field and pinch the fresh dandelion flowers off their stems. My friend Adele Dawson taught me the basic recipe and I've included a few of my own additions—Adele said a recipe was never to be followed exactly. Have fun. Take 1 cup of whole-wheat pastry flour or a mixture of brown rice, barley, and whole-wheat flours and mix in 1 teaspoon of arrowroot. Add one egg yolk, ½–1 teaspoon of your favorite herb vinegar made from brown rice or apple cider, one cup of water, a pinch of salt, kelp, or tamari, and some freshly chopped garlic. Gently stir the dry and wet

ingredients together until the consistency is similar to pan-
cake batter. Heat up safflower or canola oil in a frying pan,
dip the flower heads into the batter, and fry quickly until a
golden brown. Place them on a brown paper bag to drain.
Serve hot.

MILK THISTLE   (*Silybum marianum*) *Compositae*, Daisy Family
Other common names: Lady's milk, Mary's thistle
Parts used: Ripe seed and leaf

Milk thistle is a biennial and originated in the Mediterranean area. It is widely
cultivated in Europe because of the seeds'
numerous and effective medicinal properties. It has naturalized itself along the
northern California and southern Oregon
coast and has begun to be cultivated in
various herbalists' gardens in the United
States. Milk thistle was once grown for
food, and being the thistle it is, escaped
to various parts of the world including Africa, India, South America,
Australia, China, and the United
States.

Milk thistle prefers full sun and
well-drained soil and multiplies readily
in wild places. In my Maine gardens,
milk thistle continues to surprise me
with the places it chooses to reseed. The
large, spiny leaves are green with milky-white

Milk Thistle

veins and form a rosette the first year. In our gardens the width of
the rosette sometimes reaches three to four feet across and usually
sends up a flower stalk the first year. The familiar-looking thistle
flower waits to appear in the second year in areas where winters are
milder. The flowers grow on two-to-six-foot-high stalks and are pur-

ple with long spikes. The seeds are collected as the flower head turns fuzzy. I collect some for starting plants indoors in March. I let some reseed naturally, and I seed some into specific beds in the fall or the following spring. I feel an affinity with this plant and continue to be excited each time I see a new green and white leaf poking through the soil in the gardens.

The widespread use of the seed for various liver problems stems from the silymarin content found in the seeds of milk thistle, but not in other thistle species. Research shows silymarin helps restore healthy functioning of the liver and improves digestion when damage has occurred from drugs, alcohol, mushroom poisoning, environmental radiation, therapeutic radiation, toxic chemicals, or heavy metals. The seeds protect the liver cells from chemical damage and can help to regenerate damaged liver cells. It is an important herb to include in formulas for people with hepatitis, cirrhosis or gallbladder problems, or for anyone receiving radiation. Milk thistle is also safe for pregnant and nursing women and promotes the production of breast milk.

An effective way to take milk thistle seed is by grinding some seeds in a coffee grinder and eating 1 tablespoon, twice daily, on a regular, ongoing basis. Store a few weeks' worth of the ground seeds in your freezer and take out what you need each day. Sprinkle them on your cereal, salad, rice, or steamed vegetables. I think milk thistle seeds are an important food source for all women to use regularly to support their liver. (Pacific Botanicals sells good-quality milk thistle seeds by the pound. They are listed in the resources list.) Milk thistle seed capsules and tinctures are also available through various herb companies.

YELLOW DOCK   (*Rumex crispus*) *Polyganaceae*, Buckwheat
    Family
Other common names: Curly dock, narrow-leaved dock
Parts used: Roots, leaves, and seeds

Yellow dock is another wayside weed that commonly grows in gardens, fields, and along roadsides. The lower leaves are pointed and curly, hence the name curly dock. I prefer to gather the spring roots for tea and tincture from the first-year plants, which do not have a flower stalk. The beautiful flower stalk appears in the second year with flowers growing in a series of whorls. The stalk varies from one to five feet tall. The flowers are green in the spring and turn brown in August. Each seed is heart shaped and reminds me of fairy wings.

When yellow dock comes into your garden, consider yourself and your liver blessed. Eat the greens in soup or just steamed during the spring months. They are the first green to appear in our gardens in late April and we gather the leaves with excitement, for they signal the beginning of fresh food from the garden. The first-year roots are a healthy addition to a long-cooking soup. As you learn the valuable medicinal and nutritional properties of the so-called weeds, you will never again curse yellow dock or dandelion, but welcome them into your garden and dooryard.

Yellow dock roots and leaves have a slightly bitter taste to me, though some people claim they taste extremely bitter. They are nourishing and mildly stimulating to the liver and combine well with dandelion roots. Yellow dock roots are also mildly stimulating to the bowels and useful for constipation. It is an herb I often add into formulas for chronic skin problems such as eczema, psoriasis, and acne, along with other herbs specific for the person's situation.

Yellow dock roots combined with nettle leaves increase iron levels in the body. They are safe for pregnant and nursing women and for any woman low in iron to take two to three times a day, four to five times a week for several weeks or months.

Yellow Dock Syrup for Increasing Iron

Take 2–4 tablespoons of fresh or dried chopped yellow dock roots and place them in a pan with 2 cups of water. Simmer for twenty minutes. Strain off the herbs and place the liquid back in the pan and simmer until the liquid is half the volume, which is 1 cup. Take off the heat and immediatly dissolve 3 tablespoons of honey and 1 tablespoon of black-strap molasses into the yellow dock concentrate. Let it cool and pour into a sterilized glass jar and cover. Label and store in the refrigerator. The syrup should last for two months. Add 1 tablespoon of brandy if you want to preserve the syrup for several months. Take 1 teaspoon, four to six times a week.

Spring Tonic Soup

The following proportions are guidelines. Feel free to use whatever amounts of herbs and vegetables you have available and like.

2 onions

2–4 fresh burdock roots

¼–½ cup yellow dock roots

½ cup dandelion roots

1–2 beets

1–2 parsnips

1–2 Jerusalem artichokes

1–2 potatoes

2–3 carrots

2–4 ounces of wakame or kelp

1–3 stalks of chopped lovage

1 or more cups chopped dandelion greens

1 or more cups chopped yellow dock greens

Sauté the onion in toasted sesame oil or canola oil. Depending on how thick you prefer your soups, warm up 4–6 cups of water in a soup pot, add in all your roots, lovage, and sea vegetables and simmer for thirty to forty minutes, or until tender. Then add fresh dandelion and yellow dock greens and garlic and simmer a few more minutes. Garnish with fresh chickweed greens and chives and 2–4 cloves of chopped garlic. Mix a teaspoon of barley miso into your soup bowl for extra flavor and nourishment.

Liver Tonic

The following herbs aid in detoxifying and strengthening the liver and gallbladder. This liver tonic can help cleanse, revitalize, and protect the liver from chemical poisons and is useful to take during the recovery stage of hepatitis, cirrhosis, and alcohol and drug abuse. These herbs help heal digestive dysfunctions that accompany various liver disorders.

Dandelion roots and leaves—2 parts

Milk thistle seed—2 parts (or eat 2 Tbl, ground up, daily)

Blessed thistle leaves—1 part

Chicory root—1 part

Wild yam root—2 parts

Dose and Use: Take ¼–½ teaspoon tincture, two to three times per day after meals. As a liver tonic, use for six to eight weeks or longer if needed. For chronic liver or digestive problems, seek appropriate guidance. For a tea, simmer 4 Tbl in 1 quart of water, covered, for 20–30 mins. Take off heat, add 1 Tbl blessed thistle and steep 10 minutes.

Alcyone's Spring Tonic Tea or Tincture

A mixture of the following herbs helps to rejuvenate the body after a long winter.

Dandelion roots—2 parts

Burdock roots—1 part

Yellow dock roots—½ part

Nettle leaves—2 parts

Dose and Use: Simmer 6 tablespoons of roots together in 1 quart of water for twenty to thirty minutes, covered. Save the roots for making another batch of tea. I usually put in less water when making the second batch so the flavor will be strong. Add the nettle leaves and steep covered ten to twenty minutes. Drink 1–3 cups, four to five times a week in the spring and fall. As a tincture, take ¼–½ teaspoon, three times per day for four to six weeks in the spring and fall.

Spring Leaf and Flower Tea

This leaf and flower tea is a refreshing tea after drinking hearty root teas.

Violet leaves and flowers—2 parts

Sweet cicely leaves—2 parts

Nettle leaves—1 part

Raspberry leaves—1 part

Mint leaves—1 part

A few heartsease pansy flowers

Dose and Use: If you have a garden with any of these plants, or live in an area where violets, nettle, and raspberry grow, gather these herbs fresh each time you want to make tea. Place 10–12 tablespoons of fresh herbs, or 5–6 tablespoons of dried herbs, in 2–3 cups of cool water and let sit for a few hours, or slowly warm, covered, and let steep five to ten minutes and drink warm or cool.

Spring Tonic Vinegar

Any of the following spring greens and flowers make a nourishing and delightful vinegar: dandelion leaves and flowers, chive blossoms and greens, wild geranium leaves and flowers, mustard greens, nettle greens, wild Canada mayflower leaves, violet leaves and flowers, yellow dock leaves, lungwort leaves, coltsfoot flowers, chickweed, chicory leaves, arugula, radicchio, watercress, garlic, fresh green tips of balsam fir trees. Many of these greens can also be made into a wonderful spring salad.

Place whatever amounts of fresh herbs are available to you in a glass jar. Completely cover the herbs with organic apple cider vinegar or brown rice vinegar. Cover, preferably with a glass or plastic lid. Let sit in a sunny window for one month. Strain off the liquid through cheesecloth and compost the herbs and store the vinegar in a glass jar with a nonmetal lid in a dark, cool place for up to three years.

Herbs for the Gastrointestinal (GI) Tract

If the GI tract is weak then the body is unable to absorb nutrients and eliminate waste materials properly. This can result in various digestive problems such as diarrhea, constipation, gas, cramps, anemia, and lack of physical energy.

Nutrients from food and from emotional and spiritual sources are needed for good health. Individual nutritional needs vary throughout the world, within cultures and climates, and are affected by such things as lifestyle, physical activity, poverty, starvation, the prenatal care your mother received, and your birth and childhood experiences.

People often ask me what they can take for this particular stomachache or pain. Simple habit changes sometimes reduce and eliminate a problem without "taking something." We are so accustomed to taking something to fix us. Give yourself a few moments to sit quietly. Breathe deeply into your belly. Let your jaw and tongue relax and your shoulders drop. The more you practice this simple breathing exercise the more you will remember to call upon it when you feel stressed. The following simple practices can help some simple digestive discomforts associated with nervousness and stress disappear without the use of herbs.

- Sit while eating. How many of us eat on the go?
- In some simple way, even if for only a moment, notice that you are eating.
- Remember to breathe while eating and practice chewing your food instead of swallowing it partially chewed. This allows the saliva to do a better job at beginning the breakdown of food.
- Drinking liquids with meals dilutes the digestive enzymes, thereby inhibiting complete digestion, and can be the cause of gas and cramps. Try to drink twenty minutes prior to eating and wait a half hour or more after you have finished before drinking tea.
- Eating lighter meals at night allows the body to rest more completely while sleeping. Allowing two hours before bed-time after eating prevents food from putrifying overnight in the stomach.
- For families, mealtimes, especially the evening meal, can be challenging, with food flying around and tired or unhappy children crying. It's not always a relaxing time for the adults or older children. Perhaps the simple practice of breathing through the hard moments can help you and your family stay a bit more relaxed.

HERBS FOR INDIGESTION

Emotional stress and food habits are important factors to consider along with herbal help. Various herbs can be used for easing a stom-achache, abdominal cramping, or gas, and every herbalist has her favorites. The following tea is a favorite of mine. It can also be used before dinner and before bed to help calm and quiet children.

Belly Tea

Lemon Balm—2 parts
Linden flowers—1 part
Chamomile—2 parts

Catnip—1 part

Oatstraw—1 part

Peppermint—1 part

Dose and Use: Pour 1–2 cups of hot steaming water over 2–4 tablespoons of the tea mixture and steep, covered, for ten minutes. Drink warm before and after meals.

Chewing on a few fennel, anise, or dill seeds after a meal helps alleviate gas and a bellyache caused by a rich meal or food that did not quite agree with your digestive system. Blueberry juice is also a helpful remedy for stomach upsets.

Digest-Ease

For indigestion associated with acute stress, the following tincture can be used three times a day before meals along with addressing the deeper underlying causes.

Scullcap—2 parts

Blue vervain—1 part

Motherwort—1 part

Chamomile—1 part

Fennel seed—1 part

Dose and Use: For a child, give 2–10 drops and 25–50 drops for an adult as needed.

THE TASTE OF BITTER

Bitter tasting herbs improve slow and sluggish digestion and are especially important to take for several weeks after an infectious disease that depletes the vital force of the body. They help the body to assimilate vitamins and minerals, strengthen poor digestion due to liver-related illnesses, and stimulate the appetite.

Various kinds of stress deplete the body's vital force, which in turn adversely affects digestion and lowers the body's resistance to dis-ease. People who sit behind computers or do paperwork all day long are especially at risk of depleting their vital force because they usually overwork their minds and stress their physical bodies by sitting in one position for too long. A diet high in sugar and processed and packaged foods also weakens the digestive tract and vital life force. People who are accustomed to eating sweet-tasting foods usually do not like the taste of bitter foods and herbs. Many people today are addicted to sugar and need good ongoing support to help them understand the roots of the addiction and change their eating habits. The body needs the taste of bitter to stimulate various metabolic processes associated with the liver and digestion. People who cannot stand the taste of bitter herbs even in tincture form can take bitter herbs in capsule form. The gastric mucosa is still stimulated when bitter substances come in contact with it through bitter herbal capsules. As your digestion improves, slowly introduce bitter foods and herbs into your diet.

Bitters Tonic

Gentian root—2 parts
Blessed thistle—2 parts
Burdock root—1 part
Ginger root—1 part
Licorice root—¼ part

Dose and Use: Take as tea or tincture, twenty to thirty minutes before meals for several weeks or months. To make tea, place 6–7 tablespoons of herbs in one quart of water and simmer for thirty minutes, covered. As a tincture, take 15–30 drops. These herbs are an excellent tonic for the recuperative stage of any illness where digestive problems are present, including anorexia, and for people whose digestive systems have been weakened due to long-term use of alcohol or drugs.

An herbal elixir made in West Germany, Swedish Bitters, is widely available in health food stores and food co-ops and is an excellent bitters tonic. I also make a bitters tonic for Avena Botanicals that works well.

Overactive Digestion

The following herbs help overcome an overactive digestive system, soothe the mucous membranes of the digestive tract, reduce excess acidity, and ease gastritis, nausea, and heartburn. They are helpful to use when traveling and eating foods to which you are unaccustomed, and are also safe for pregnant women to use to relieve nausea.

Meadowsweet flowers—2 parts

Peach leaves—1 part

Chamomile flowers—2 parts

Fennel seed—1 part

Dose and Use: As a digestive aid, take a tincture or tea twenty minutes before eating. For heartburn and digestive upsets, take after meals. For a child, 2–10 drops of tincture or ¼ cup tea. For an adult, 25–50 drops of tincture or ½–1 cup tea.

One of the most memorable and peaceful mealtime experiences I have had was at a meditation retreat led by the Vietnamese Buddhist monk and teacher, Thich Nhat Hanh. Six hundred people ate in silence. Quite remarkable and wonderful. A designated person would ring a special bell called the Mindfulness Bell every now and then throughout the meals, reminding us to come back to our breath and to the present moment. We would all stop eating, breathe three times, and then pick up our forks and begin eating again. The practice of using the Mindfulness Bell works well with children and families and even in the workplace at different intervals throughout a day to remind everyone to breathe and to notice that they are alive.

DIARRHEA AND CONSTIPATION

Diarrhea can be the result of such things as nervousness, overexcitement, allergic reactions to food, an improperly functioning digestive system, or an infection in the gut. Seek appropriate help if there is mucus or blood in the stools, if fever is present, or if the condition persists longer than twenty-four hours for a baby, or if the child or adult (or animal) becomes dehydrated.

Constipation can be caused by eating too much refined food, poor digestion, feeling angry or uptight, wearing constricting clothing, lack of exercise, or the lack of bowel muscle tone due to overuse of laxatives. When the body is constipated, too much water and waste materials are absorbed from the colon back into the body, setting the body up for various dis-eases. The body is unable to assimilate nutrients when either diarrhea or constipation is present. If either of these conditions is chronic, seek appropriate help from your health care provider. Changes in bowel habits that persist can be signs of a serious disease and need attention.

Diarrhea Remedy

Blackberry root bark, the roots of wild geranium, and meadowsweet flowers are excellent herbs for helping diarrhea. A tea made from marshmallow root and cinnamon bark and/or an infusion of lady's mantle leaves, raspberry leaves, and blackberry leaves can also be helpful. If cramping is present, ginger root, peppermint, or chamomile can be added. Take the tea and/or tincture every one to two hours until symptoms subside.

A Constipation Remedy

Along with addressing the underlying causes and supporting the appropriate systems in the body that are stressed with herbs and food and lifestyle changes, such as eating more fiber, drinking more water, and excercising regularly, the following herbs can be helpful.

Soak 1–2 teaspoons of psyllium seed in one cup of hot water for two hours. Add freshly squeezed lemon and a touch of honey and drink before going to bed. Drink in the morning if needed. Some people have found drinking a cup of warm water upon rising in the morning also helps. People with chronic constipation may also find help in drinking a tea or taking a tincture of the following herbs three times a week for one to three weeks.

Dandelion root—2 parts

Yellow dock root—1 part

Angelica root—2 parts

Burdock root—1 part

Ginger root—1 part

Licorice root—½ part

Dose and Use: Place 7–8 tablespoons of herbs in 1 quart of water and simmer, covered, for thirty minutes. Drink warm as needed. As a tincture, take 25–50 drops as needed.

ANOREXIA NERVOSA

Anorexia nervosa is a form of self-starvation and occurs most commonly among young women. Some signs to note include being overly anxious about weight gain, poor body image and low self-esteem, unusual patterns of handling food, severe weight loss, and amenorrhoea. Anorexia is a serious form of starving oneself that can lead to death.

Many women have used food at some time to comfort themselves or deny their feelings, especially women who have experienced some form of sexual abuse. The underlying pain needs to be addressed with appropriate ongoing support, besides using herbs to support the various systems in the body that are out of balance. Seek herbal care from a sensitive and experienced herbalist or health care provider to help design herbal formulas specific for the individual. Medical evaluation and counseling is necessary for severely ill people, who risk various health complications and electrolyte abnormalities.

The following two remedies support the nervous and digestive system through the use of nerve tonics and herbs that relax the nervous system and bitter herbs that stimulate appetite and improve overall metabolism.

Tea

Oatstraw—2 parts

Lemon verbena—1 part

Lemon Balm—2 parts

Sweet marjoram—2 parts

Lavender—1 part

Calendula—1 part

Dose and Use: Add 5–6 teaspoons of herbs to 1 cup of hot water and steep ten to fifteen minutes, covered. Drink 2–3 cups per day.

Tincture

Gentian root—2 parts

Blessed thistle—2 parts

St. Johnswort—2 parts

Blue vervain—1 part

Catnip—1 part

Chamomile—1 part

Dose and Use: Take tincture, 25–50 drops, twice a day before meals.

Groups providing information about anorexia are listed under Women's Health Resources at the back of this book.

LIVING IN HARMONY WITH THE SEASONS

This chart is offered as a basic guideline for cleansing & rebuilding the body during the different seasons. It is not meant to be used in a rigid way — the herbs and foods listed can be used at different times during the year depending on your body's needs.

Seasons	Organs	Out of Balance	Taste	Supportive Herbs	Nourishing Foods
Spring Wood element	Liver, Gall bladder	frustrated, blocked creativity, anger	sour	Dandelion roots & greens, yellow dock roots & green, nettle tea & steamed nettles, violet leaf tea & salad, wild mustard greens & other edible wild greens	Quinoa, barley, rye, lemon water, kim-chi, daikon, arugula, carrots, beets, cabbage, broccoli, wakame, arame, kelp, dulse, chives, umeboshi plums
Summer Fire	Heart, Small Intestines	over-excited, over-works, inability to relax	bitter	Blessed thistle, chamomile, hawthorn flowers, motherwort, mustard greens & other bitter greens, raspberry leaves, rosemary, yarrow	Pot-boiled brown rice, quinoa, corn, summer garden vegetables, salads, dulse, kelp, nori, local fruit, especially strawberries
Late Summer Earth	Spleen-Pancreas, Stomach	scattered, mood swings, overwhelmed, stuck in a rut	sweet	Anise-hyssop, codonopsis root*, ginseng, goldenrod, hawthorn berries, licorice root, marshmallow root	Corn, millet, sweet-tasting vegetables, onions, summer squash, blueberries, blackberries, raspberries, early apples & pears, melons, arame, dulse, kelp, miso soup
Fall metal	Lungs, Large Intestine	Grief, despair, depression, hypercritical	spicy	Astragalus root*, elderberries, garlic, ginger, hawthorn berries, hyssop, mullein, schizandra berries*, siberian ginseng	Brown rice, winter squash, yams, kale, collards, root vegetables, chard, onions, leeks, miso soup, wakame, hijiki, kelp, dulse, apples, pears
Winter water	Kidneys, Bladder	Fear, anxiety, paranoia, terror	salty	Astragalus root*, burdock root, dong quai root*, echinacea root, garlic, ginger, sacred basil, siberian ginseng, usnea	Brown rice, buckwheat, winter squash, root vegetables, kale, collards, arame, kelp, hijiki, dulse, miso soup

* Chinese herbs

6

Menstrual Wisdom

The healing available to contemporary women through our blood cycle is an instinctual release of what is within us. Our willingness to face the dark is the key to our own development. What we're afraid of is actually the treasure at the center of our being, the female source energy from which we have so long been severed.[1]

—VICKI NOBLE

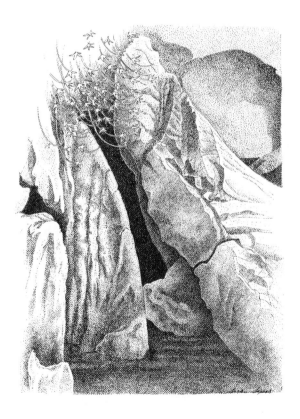

Various cultures once honored menstruating women and associated women's monthly bleeding with the sacred powers of the moon. The moon symbolized woman's deep unconscious being, which held divine knowledge about the cycles of life and death. Most women raised in modern-day cultures are not taught to regard their bodies, their menstrual cycles, and their connection to nature as something sacred. How many of us were encouraged to gently massage our bellies and admire and touch our vaginas and our blood when we first began bleeding? Many women today flush their blood and disposable tampons down the toilet with little understanding of their body's monthly cycles.

Whether or not we give birth to a baby, we women carry an understanding of the mysteries of birth, life, death, and renewal deep within us. The energy in our wombs and the cyclical nature of our hormones creates internal changes that are unique and deeply personal for each woman. Our monthly cycles wax and wane like the moon's phases. The ebbing and flowing of our energy resembles the ocean's tides.

Women's understanding of divine consciousness is centered in our wombs. Prepatriarchal cultures knew this and honored the female body. Marija Gimbutas, an archaeologist of Lithuanian origin and author of several books including *The Language of the Goddess* and *The Civilization of the Goddess*, documents female-centered civilizations of Old Europe. Both books are filled with photos and drawings of ancient female figurines with large hips, bellies, breasts, and buttocks, illustrating how revered women were during the Goddess worshipping times. Patricia Reis writes in her book, *Through The Goddess: A Woman's Way of Healing,*

> These Great Goddess figures embody the notion of a complete, self-fulfilling, self-sustaining, and self-generating femaleness that does not demand a bloody sacrifice from the male. She is an image that is complete unto herself. For this reason she is impor-

tant as a reminder and an expres-
sion of female wholeness.[2]

"The Bird-Headed Snake Goddess," (4000
B.C.E.) from pre-historic Egypt. A grounding
and powerful stance, reminding women how
strong and beautiful we are. This statue is rooted in
the earth and at the same time connected to the
sky. Her snake-like shape honors the interconnectedness of all life forms. (Drawn from a photograph from *The Heart of the Goddess: Art, Myth
and Meditations of the World's Sacred Feminine,*
by Hallie Iglehart Austen, Berkeley: Wingbow
Press, 1990, p. 9.)

Gimbutas traces the Goddess tradition back to the Paleolithic period (approximately thirty thousand years ago), through
the Neolithic time (around nine thousand
years ago), through the transition into a patriarchal society (five
thousand years ago), and into the present. She spent several
decades excavating, researching, and piecing together the extensive
information she thoroughly presents in her books. *The Language of
the Goddess* and *The Civilization of the Goddess* are especially valuable books for women who are rediscovering their Old European
roots and spiritual heritages.

I was fortunate to have met and corresponded with Marija
Gimbutas about herbs during the last year of her life. I visited her at
her home in Topanga, California, two days before she went into the
hospital for the last time in January of 1994. I sat next to her bed
and held her hand. I reminded Marija of a conversation we had
shared at an earlier date about her mother telling her when she was
young that she would do work that would prevent illness. Indeed,
Marija's work has profoundly helped contemporary women create
healthier relationships with their bodies by reintroducing the

ancient Goddess figurines and numerous other
female symbols into our consciousness.
The Sanskrit word *yoni* means vulva,

Sprouting seeds and plants were carved on figurines
in the vulva areas in various cultures of Old Europe
during the 5th and 6th millennia B.C.E. Also note
the crescent or bull horns (which Marija Gimbutas
spoke of as being shaped like fallopian tubes) below
the neck. (Drawn from a drawing in *The Language of
the Goddess* by Marija Gimbutas. London: Thames
and Hudson, 1989, p. 168.)

womb, temple, sanctuary, place of birth. In various locations around the world, yoni shaped
objects and womb shaped caves have been found.
I visited a sacred *dakini** pool in Nepal, which has
a natural spring running out of vaginally shaped rocks. This rock
formation is visited monthly by Buddhists. Near the spring is a sim-
iliar rock formation with a carved image of the elephant deity
Ganesh next to it. These rocks are covered with red tika powder
and flowers—offerings left by Hindu pilgrims who visit the site
monthly. In Glastonbury, England, a pilgrimage spot for Western-
ers, red iron oxide colors a running stream in an ancient Goddess
worshipping pool, symbolizing the female blood mysteries.

Women's bodies, intuition, feelings, and connection to nature
are not recognized and valued by the postindustrial world. Menstrual blood is considered disgusting, unclean, and smelly. These

Dakini represents one of the most important, potent, and dynamic
images/ideas/symbols within all of Tantric Buddhism. Yet, precisely owing to such
dynamism and power, it is impossible to pin it down or to limit it to a single defi-
nition—prophetess, protectress, fairy, sprite, witch, inspirer, goddess with magical
powers, she who goes in the sky.[3]

types of antifemale messages wound our psyches. It is not surprising that many of us experience dis-ease in the organs we associate with giving life and pleasure: breasts, vagina, uterus, heart, stomach, and digestive tract. Recent medical statistics show that over 60 percent of women in the United States experience premenstrual discomfort, over 50 percent will have hysterectomies, 40 percent have uterine fibroids, one in eight women will develop breast cancer, and a growing percentage suffer from chronic vaginitis, urinary tract infections, endometriosis, and menopausal difficulties. In the United States, one in three women is the victim of rape and one in four is the survivor of sexual abuse.[4]

Western culture, to an alarming extent, worships money and values a fast-paced, superficial lifestyle. Our bodies ask something different of us when we bleed. We are closer to the rhythms and whispers of the Earth and moon during this part of our cycle. It is a time for deeper dreaming, resting, and healing. Many women find that slowing down and listening to what their bodies want when they bleed makes a tremendous difference in easing or eliminating the discomforts they experienced in the past. This is not possible yet for most women today, given the enormous responsibilities they shoulder.

I believe that understanding our bodies' natural rhythms and menstrual cycles can once again teach us to love ourselves, help us to feel how precious our lives are, and give us strength and courage to create a peaceful and just world. Women deeply understand how to nurture all life forms. As we change our misconceptions about menstruation and women, we shake up the established institutions whose negative beliefs about women's bodies have been wounding and killing us.

A SIGH

A sigh
I finally give in to,
lay my body down
and do nothing
but feel its weight
settle against the ground

Grateful,
my body reminds me of this quiet pleasure
—rest

We breathe
slowly,
together
again.

—Nancy Devine

NUTRITION FOR THE MENSTRUAL CYCLE

Nutritious food is a basic need for maintaining and supporting our bodies. Keep in mind as you read the following information that hunger and poverty affect millions of people in the United States and around the world. Issues surrounding food, overeating, and an overemphasis on being healthy also present challenges for many Western women.

Changes in diet can prevent and relieve various pains and emotional stresses associated with the menstrual cycle. Excessive amounts of alcohol, caffeine, nicotine, sugar, white flour products, and red meats aggravate hormonal changes, decrease nutritional absorption, and weaken the liver. Alcohol, caffeine, and nicotine

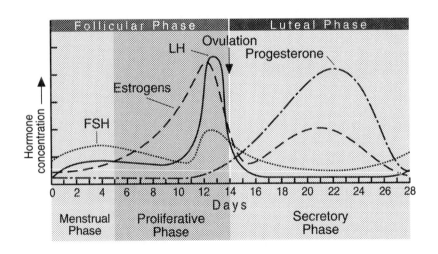

leach iron and other important minerals and vitamins from the body, which, over time, leaves the body in a weakened and vulnerable state. Blood-sugar levels stabilize when more whole grains (brown rice, millet, barley, oats, amaranth) and less flours (even whole grain flours) are eaten. This evens out drastic mood swings and feelings of depression.

A healthy liver is especially important to women for many reasons. The liver helps convert estrogen to a harmless metabolite, which then balances the estrogen-progesterone levels. Many menstrual and menopausal difficulties lessen or disappear when hormonal levels become balanced and health is improved. A diet low in meat, dairy, and other fatty foods and rich in dark green leafy vegetables, whole grains, and nourishing herbs helps the liver be less congested and better able to process female sex hormones.

Regular movement, such as walking, running, dancing, yoga, stacking firewood, or whatever you prefer or are physically able to do, stimulates the liver's microsomal enzymes and increases the level of endorphins in our brains. Endorphins lighten our moods and raise our spirits. Moving our bodies lets us know ourselves more completely, strengthens our muscles and internal boundaries, and relieves tension. Many women are too hard on themselves about "exercising." Move in ways that feel nourishing to you and that you can incorporate into your life without disrupting your personal rhythm.

SUPPLEMENTS

Major nutritional needs for the first part of the menstrual cycle, bleeding through ovulation, include sufficient Vitamin B6, iron, and protein.

Vitamin B6

Vitamin B6 assists the liver in breaking down reproductive hormones. It aids in relieving mood swings, irritability, fluid retention, breast tenderness, sugar cravings, and fatigue. Vitamin B6 is depleted by the use of oral contraceptives, fasting, radiation, pregnancy, and lactation. *Foods containing vitamin B6*: rice bran, kale, buckwheat flour, navy beans, lentils, lima beans, pinto beans, black-eyed peas, brown rice, broccoli, asparagus, brussels sprouts, beet greens, sunflower seeds, sweet potatoes, cauliflower, and leeks.[5]

If you choose to take a vitamin B6 supplement, take in a B-complex vitamin.

Iron

Iron-rich foods are especially important to eat during menstruation and the two weeks following because iron is lost through menstrual blood. Special attention needs to be given to iron intake during pregnancy, nursing, and before and after any surgery. Iron is depleted by black teas, coffee, chocolate, enemas, and lack of high quality protein in the diet.

Some iron-rich herbs and foods: wild or organically grown stinging nettle leaves, taken as a tea, 2–4 cups of tea per day, eaten as a steamed vegetable (use spring-picked leaves), or taken in tincture form one to three times per day; fresh parsley; watercress; dandelion greens; yellow dock roots; black-strap molasses; raisins; seaweeds; miso; ground, unhulled sesame seeds; and steamed, dark leafy vegetables such as kale, collards, turnip, mustard, and beet greens.

Protein and Carbohydrates

Estrogen is produced during the follicular stage (menstruation until ovulation) of our menstrual cycle (refer to chart on page 100). Estrogen levels peak just before ovulation. The body produces more protein during this phase and therefore needs adequate protein to ensure overall nutrition. A regular diet with combinations of beans, nuts and seeds, grains, and dark leafy green vegetables offers balanced sources of protein and fiber. Pregnant and nursing mothers and women doing strenuous physical labor or outdoor adventures require more protein.

Higher levels of progesterone circulate in our bloodstream after ovulation occurs. Just before bleeding begins, progesterone levels drop off. Many women say they feel this "hormone drop" and suddenly feel tired, irritable, and unsociable. Recognizing how we feel when our hormones change helps us know how to care for ourselves during these transitions.

Progesterone levels are connected to carbohydrate metabolism. Many women experience sugar cravings and feelings of depression and fatigue just before bleeding begins because the brain is not receiving enough glucose. The brain sends out messages that it is starving for sugar. Symbolically, a woman may also be starving for emotional or spiritual nourishment, rest, and a quiet home.

Foods high in complex carbohydrates, such as whole grains and beans, offer the body a steadier supply of glucose and prevent the sugar rush and crash that can occur after eating excess amounts of sugar. Some women may find eating smaller and more frequent meals during the last stage of their cycle helps to stabilize blood-sugar levels and prevent constipation.

The energy in the last phase of our menstrual cycle is slower. The digestive system slows down. This can result in either constipation or diarrhea. Eating fewer varieties and smaller amounts of food supports the hormonal changes and allows our bodies to focus on internal, emotional concerns instead of putting out energy to digest food.

Calcium

Calcium levels decrease after ovulation because estrogen levels are lower. Many women find eating foods high in calcium throughout the month prevents menstrual cramps and pain and helps maintain normal muscle tone. Equal amounts of magnesium to calcium or at least half the amount of magnesium to calcium is needed to assist the body in absorbing calcium.

Dairy food is not an ideal source of calcium or protein because of its high fat and protein content. Excess dairy can cause diarrhea and intestinal cramping and gas. It also increases fluid retention and bloating due to its sodium content. However, it's important to note that a little butter is healthier than margarine, even soy margarine. Margarine is a transfatty acid, and the body does not know what to do with this type of fatty acid. Margarine is made by heating vegetable oil to extremely high temperatures and blowing hydrogen into the bonds in the fat. This is what is meant by hydrogenated fats. Try to avoid foods with hydrogenated fats listed on the label.

Calcium is depleted by lack of weight-bearing exercise, by coffee, sugar, salt, alcohol, cortisone, and enemas. A high fat and protein diet inhibits calcium absorption. Excess fat also interferes with healthy functioning of the liver, heart, intestines, and bowels. High salt intake increases calcium loss through the urine. Carbonated beverages deplete calcium from the body because of their high phosphoric acid content. Average Americans consume three to six cans of soda per day.

Foods containing calcium: collard greens; black-strap molasses; ground, unhulled sesame seeds; lightly steamed bok choy; kale; mustard greens; broccoli; tofu; carob flour; rutabagas; and sea vegetables.[6]

The recommended daily dosage of calcium is 800 milligrams.

Herbs containing calcium: raspberry leaves, oatstraw, horsetail, nettles, borage leaves, dandelion greens.

Magnesium

Magnesium decreases menstrual cramps and premenstrual sugar cravings by assisting in glucose metabolism. Magnesium is depleted by alcohol, enemas, and some pharmaceutical drugs.

Foods containing magnesium: beets; beet greens; black-eyed peas; white beans; lima beans; red beans; buckwheat; tofu; turnip greens; collard greens; cornmeal; millet; dandelion greens; lentils; cashews; mustard greens; brown rice; peas; oatmeal; sweet potatoes; brussels sprouts; kale; almonds; ground, unhulled sesame seeds; parsnips; turnips; corn; broccoli; cauliflower; barley; summer squash; carrots; celery; cabbage; sunflower seeds; parsley; and dulse.[7]

Potassium

Low levels of potassium can also be a cause of fatigue. Potassium helps regulate the fluid balance of the body and stimulates intestinal movements. A regular bowel movement prevents the body from reabsorbing waste products and fluids that need to be eliminated from the body. Constipation can lead to fatigue, weight gain, skin problems, poor nutrient assimilation, and other health complications. Potassium is depleted by diuretics, vomiting, diarrhea, enemas, coffee, sugar, salt, and alcohol.

Foods containing potassium: green beans; beet greens; broccoli; brussels sprouts; carrots; celery; Swiss chard; collard greens; kale; mustard greens; parsley; parsnips; potatoes; spinach; squash; yams; walnuts; ground, unhulled sesame seeds; sunflower seeds; apples; oranges; cantaloupes; ripe dates; figs; grapefruit; lemons; raisins; kelp; and dulse.

Herbs containing potassium: Chamomile, watercress, parsley, nettles, dandelion roots and greens, alfalfa, chicory roots and greens, and plantain leaves.

TO SLEEP AND DREAM

Deep relaxing and resting regularly is necessary for restoring vitality and peace. Resting before and during our menstrual flow supports our body's slower pace. When we resist our body's natural rhythms, imbalances and discomforts occur. Artificial light and lack of exposure to the sun and moon also upset the balance of the menstrual cycle. Spending time outside in the moonlight is a wonderful ritual to bring into your life. Observe the moon as she waxes and wanes, and chart how your body feels during the different moon phases. Sleep with your curtains open to the moonlight or even sleep outside. If you live in the city, make a weekly or monthly pilgrimage to a place where you can be in the moonlight. Keep a special book next to your bed for recording your dreams.

HERBS FOR THE MENSTRUAL CYCLE

Various herbs support our bodies' changes and natural rhythms. They help support and nourish the hormonal system, relieve various discomforts and pain associated with the menstrual cycle, and strengthen specific organs and functions in the body. They may be used singly or in combinations. The specific herbs or combinations you choose are dependent on your personal energy and/or connection to particular herbs. As you make friends with different herbs, you will come to use certain ones more often than others.

In the following section, the individual herbs are listed before the formulas. The art of using one herb at a time is the basic foundation for learning how to use herbs in combinations. If herbs are new to you, read about their properties from various sources. Study books written by people who have plenty of hands-on experience using medicinal plants. Spend time outside with plants. Sit near them. Talk with them. Listen for what they have to say. Make contact with other herbalists living nearby. Let yourself have fun.

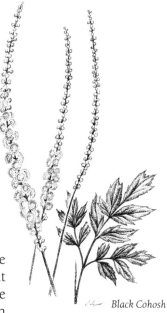

BLACK COHOSH   (*Cimicifuga racemosa*) *Ranunculaceae*, Buttercup Family
Other common names: Rattleweed, black snakeroot, rattletop, bugbane, bugwort, fairywand
Part used: Root. Dig in the spring or fall when the flower stalk is dried and rattling. Perhaps this wonderfully helpful plant will lead you to her with the soft sound of her rattle, moving in the breeze.

Black cohosh grows wild in the rich soil of hardwood forests throughout the Appalachians, from New York State south to Georgia, and from southern

Black Cohosh

Ontario to Arkansas. People also cultivate black cohosh in their gardens for its three-to-seven-foot tall white flower spike, which is a spectacular sight. I brought some roots back from North Carolina and planted them in our gardens. Much to my delight, after three years of settling in they now flower in late June through late July. The seed pods contain hard, dry seeds in late autumn and rattle in the wind. Some people say the sound of the seeds rattling is like a rattlesnake's rattle, earning it the nickname rattleweed or rattletop. Black cohosh's leaves are sharply toothed, divided into three. The leaflets are terminal with three lobes, the middle lobe being the largest.

I especially enjoy being in the western mountains of North Carolina in the springtime when the dogwood and shad trees awaken the mountainsides with their lacy white flowers. Spring arrives in North Carolina long before it does in Maine, and many times my root-digging pilgrimages to these southern mountains have been my antidote to cabin fever.

Native American women have used black cohosh root for a variety of health conditions and passed on their knowledge to interested settlers. Black cohosh root is a strong antispasmodic herb and is very effective for easing ovarian pain and uterine cramps, before and during menstruation. It is an excellent remedy to take as needed for relieving the dull, dragging muscular pain that sometimes occurs at the onset of menstruation.

Black cohosh restores tone to the uterus and reproductive organs. It helps bring on a delayed menses by stimulating the uterus and by improving blood circulation to the pelvic area. A late or irregular period can be caused by hormonal imbalances, general body weakness, pelvic congestion, or atony of the reproductive organs (which may be the result of surgery, a prolapsed uterus, or previous pregnancies or miscarriages).

Recent research shows that black cohosh root contains estrogenlike substances and may be used to help increase estrogen levels in the body for menstruating and menopausal women whose estrogen levels are low.[8] Black cohosh is an herb I commonly combine with other herbs for a general menopause tonic. Refer to chapter 10 for more information on menopause.

Black cohosh helps relax the uterus and assists in a slow and difficult labor. It encourages irregular or weak contractions to become more regular and effective and, because of its influence on the nervous system, calms an overly anxious or excited woman in labor. Black cohosh can be given as a tincture or in homeopathic form to a woman after she has given birth to ease any afterpains and to quiet the nervous system.

Black and blue cohosh in combination with other herbs can help complete a miscarriage. Seek appropriate assistance and support. If you are working with a health care provider who is knowledgeable in herbal medicine, call upon her guidance and loving support to help you through this passage.

Black cohosh also relieves muscular, bronchial, and asthmatic spasms. It eases acute chronic coughs, abdominal spasms, and any nervous tension that accompanies these conditions. After a friend of mine broke seven ribs in an accident a few years back, the muscles around her rib cage began to spasm, causing her acute pain for two days. In just twenty minutes after taking a tincture of equal parts of black cohosh and crampbark, the spasms ended and she was finally able to rest comfortably. Black cohosh is very useful in treating rheumatic pains, sciatica, neuralgia, rheumatoid arthritis, and osteoarthritis.

Black cohosh combined with ginkgo leaves can be effective in lessening ringing in the ears caused by exposure to loud, continuous noises. My neighbor, who is a professional flutist, suffered from tinnitus, ringing in the ear, for years, and after taking black cohosh tincture for a few weeks was convinced of the effectiveness of herbal medicine because of the help he received.

BLUE COHOSH   (*Caulophyllum thalictroides*) *Berberidaceae*, Barberry Family
Other common names: Blue ginseng, yellow ginseng, blue berry cohosh, blue berry root, papoose root
Part used: Root. Dig in the early spring when the leaves first unfurl and are recognizable, or later in the fall just as the leaves begin to die back.

Blue cohosh grows in rich, moist soil under hardwood trees in higher mountain elevations. It can be found growing from New England south to the Carolinas, westward to Arkansas, and north to the Canadian border. Blue cohosh is a perennial, grows to three feet in height, and has two to three large compound leaves growing on a smooth stem with a bluish color. The leaflets are rounded and look like lace to me and have a resemblance to meadow rue (*Thalictrum dioicum*). The flowers are tiny, greenish yellow in color, grow in terminal clusters, and form a blue berry in the fall.

Naturalist and author Doug Elliot first identified blue and black cohosh plants for me in the early 1980s in the North Carolina mountains. The peculiar smell of the freshly dug roots of the blue cohosh is one I especially like. I have fond memories of different outings we have shared collecting these roots, nibbling on various wild foods, and exchanging stories.

Knowledge of this plant comes to us from Native American women. Blue cohosh is an effective uterine tonic, nourishing and revitalizing the tissue of the uterus following pregnancy, a miscarriage or abortion, hysterectomy, or other abdominal surgery, after coming off the pill or other hormone-related drugs, and for any uterine weakness due to a chronic inflamed condition. It is an excellent herb to take in combination with other herbs for regulating the menstrual cycle and for reducing painful menstrual cramps over time. It is also an herb I add to formulas for endometriosis, chlamydia, and cervical dysplasia (now referred to as CIN).

Blue cohosh is often called upon during childbirth to promote effective contractions and ease labor pain. Some midwives use blue and black cohosh together to encourage regular and coordinated labor contractions. A tincture is more effective than a water-based tea since the active ingredients of both blue and black cohosh are not water soluble. Equal parts of blue and black cohosh tincture can be mixed and 40–60 drops of tincture given every hour until contractions are even and strong. Two parts blue cohosh to one part spikenard is used by some midwives when the cervix is one-half dilated and labor is slow or has stopped. Give two doses of tincture in a one-half hour period. Blue cohosh given after birth can help deliver a retained placenta and stop bleeding because it helps the uterus to clamp down without causing the cervix to close down. It is also a good herb for easing afterpains.

Some midwives recommend that women use blue cohosh tincture, once a day, starting two to three weeks before their delivery date to give the uterus some final toning, thus helping labor be smoother and less painful. Some herbalists recommend making tincture from dried root as the fresh root can be too irritating to the body.

Note: Blue cohosh can lower blood pressure. Blue and black cohosh should be avoided by pregnant women until the last month of pregnancy.

CHASTEBERRY   (*Vitex agnus-castus*) *Verbenaceae*, Verbena
    Family
Other common names: Hemp tree, cloister pepper, monk's pepper,
    chaste lamb, Abraham's balm
Part used: Fresh or dried berries, collected in the fall

Chasteberries received their name because the berries were used as a food spice in monasteries throughout the Roman Empire to decrease the monks' sexual desires. I prefer to call this herb *vitex* because the word chaste has negative connotations for many people. Some herbalists claim that vitex has a different action in women's bodies than in men's. For women, vitex appears to replenish the body's life energy, or vitality, and increase feelings of exuberance.

Vitex is one of the first herbs I call upon for women who are experiencing various kinds of premenstrual, menstrual, and menopausal difficulties. It helps restore hormonal balance and regulate an irregular or short menstrual cycle. Some herbalists report that the berries are most effective when taken consistently over three to six months or longer for easing premenstrual and menopausal depression, anxiety, and mood swings, and for eliminating breast tenderness and water retention.

The berries regulate the proper levels of progesterone and estrogen by affecting two pituitary hormones, FSH (follicle-stimulating hormone) and LH (luteinizing hormone).[9] Various uncomfortable symptoms such as depression, extreme irritability, breast tenderness, heavy bleeding, water retention, and acne can arise when estrogen levels are too high. Daily use of vitex berries over three to six months helps balance hormone levels and reduce or eliminate these symptoms, unless other health problems are involved.

I recommend this herb, often in combination with other herbs, for women coming off the pill; following an abortion, miscarriage, or pregnancy; for women who wish to become pregnant; for women whose hormone levels have been adversely affected by traveling or by the overuse of antibiotics, other drugs, alcohol, or nicotine; for women with irregular menstrual cycles; for women with cysts; and for women whose joy for life feels low.

If you wish to learn more about vitex refer to a small booklet called *Vitex*, written by herbalist and botanist Christopher Hobbs, available through bookstores and Avena Botanicals.

CRAMPBARK   (*Viburnum trilobum* or *opulus*) *Caprifoliaceae*, Honeysuckle Family
Other common names: Highbush cranberry, white dogwood, snowball tree, guelder rose
Part used: Outer and inner bark, gathered in the spring when the sap is rising or in autumn when the leaves are falling from the branches.

Crampbark is a shrub that can grow up to twelve feet. It is a wonderful addition to a hedge-row. The leaves are hairy on their underside and resemble a maple leaf with three to five lobes. The white flowers form a rounded head and bloom in June in my yard. Red berries appear in the fall and are considered poisonous to eat when unripe. Even birds avoid eating them. The red berries covered with snow are a pretty sight in the winter. Crampbark is easy to plant and requires little care. I planted seven small shrubs that were two feet tall next to my garden four years ago and they are doing well.

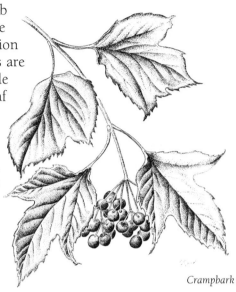

Crampbark

I gather the bark from stands of crampbark that are several years old and overcrowded. You can often find good-sized shrubs around old foundations. I carefully prune overcrowded branches with a small pruning saw, never taking bark from the main trunks, and then scrape the bark off with a sharp pocketknife. The outer and inner layers come off easily. Spring-gathered inner bark is a vibrant green color and tastes bitter. You can tincture the bark fresh or lay it on screens to dry.

This shrub is appropriately named, as it is effective for easing ovarian and uterine cramps before and during menstruation. Crampbark helps relax muscle tension and spasms in the uterus and other muscles in the body. It is especially effective for lessening lower back pain that extends down into the thighs when menstruation begins. Drink ¼ cup of tea or take 20–40 drops of tincture every half hour until cramping and pain cease. Crampbark in combination with wild yam root is useful for gastrointestinal pain and spasms. For menstrual cramps that are severe, crampbark combined with valerian root can be helpful.

Crampbark also helps relieve pain and spasms after giving birth. Follow the above suggested doses until pain subsides. I have also used crampbark in combination with false unicorn root and wild yam root as a preventative for women who have a history of miscarriages (refer to chapter 7).

DONG QUAI OR TANG KUEI (*Angelica sinensis*) *Umbelliferae*,
   Carrot Family
Other common names: Dan Gui
Part used: Root. Available in Chinese herb stores either as whole
   roots that have been sliced, steamed, and dried, or as dried
   whole roots, or heads or tails.

Angelica sinensis is indigenous to mainland China and can be cultivated in the United States. Dong Quai is a perennial that grows three to four feet tall. The umbel type flowers have nine to thirteen radial segments with lots of tiny flowers. The leaf stalk has a prominent sheath, characteristic of the *Angelica* genus, and the leaves are oval shaped, sharply toothed, and divided into threes.[10]

I am particularly fond of growing *Angelica archangelica* because of its name *angelica*, reminding me of the help and guidance the angelic realm offers gardeners. The *archangelica* species prefers a shady spot and usually grows six feet high in my gardens. Though its medicinal qualities differ from Dong Quai's properties, I mention it here for interested gardeners to further investigate.

Dong Quai has a sweet and unusually thick pungent taste and is warming and moistening to the body. It nourishes the blood, improves blood circulation throughout the pelvic area, and helps with constipation. An excellent remedy for women who are anemic, weak, or who have recently given birth to take for one to four months, or longer, if needed. Dong Quai helps prevent postpartum infections and assists in bringing energy back into the body.

Some women experience painful menses due to poor circulation and congestion in the pelvic area. Dong Quai increases circulation and nutrients to the uterus when taken daily over a few weeks or months, helping to eliminate menstrual cramps and pain.

When used as a daily tonic for one to three months or longer, the irritability and drastic mood swings some women experience premenstrually and during menopause diminish. The root can bring on menstruation after a short or long absence, even out an irregular menstrual cycle, promote fertility, and ease menopausal changes. Dong Quai also protects the liver from chemicals and toxins.

Note: Avoid use during pregnancy, or if your menstrual flow is excessive or your blood does not clot easily. Do not use if experiencing abdominal congestion and bloating, or if you have endometriosis or fibroids.

FALSE UNICORN ROOT *(Chamaelirium luteum) Lilaceaea,* Lily
   Family
Other common names: Helonias root, fairy wand, blazing star,
   starwort, devil's bit, dwarf lily, drooping starwort
Part used: Spring-or fall-dug roots; dry for tea, fresh or dried for a
   tincture

False unicorn root grows in moist meadows, bogs, thickets, and woods from Massachusetts to Michigan, and south to Florida. It is on the endangered plant list in some states, so be sure to check first before harvesting. The female and male flowers are small, white, and grow on separate stalks. The female flower spike is shorter and straighter than the male flower, and blunt at the tip. The male flower spike tapers at the end and droops, hence one of its common names is drooping starwort. I have only seen this plant in flower once, in the western North Carolina mountains in late April. The flowering plant was quite magical to come upon and I smiled to myself imagining a fairy using this flower for a wand.

The root is wonderful medicine for strengthening and toning the uterus and the whole reproductive system. False unicorn contains estrogen precursors that help balance the

False Unicorn root

hormonal system's production of hormones. It is an effective remedy for easing ovarian pain and dryness in the vagina and for bringing on a delayed or absent menses.

False unicorn can be taken for several weeks to help restore strength and tone to the uterus after childbirth, an abortion, miscarriage, surgery, infection in the pelvic area, extended use of drugs or alcohol, or for promoting fertility. It is a supportive herb for a woman experiencing hormonal changes during menopause or one who has had a hysterectomy. Women with ovarian cysts or endometriosis may take false unicorn root with other herbs over several weeks to increase circulation to the pelvic area. (Refer to formulas in next chapter for specifics on ovarian cysts and endometriosis.) Women healing from sexual abuse experiences may find the root helpful in restoring feelings of strength and vitality in their womb area when taken a few times a week.

False unicorn root is a good remedy for women with prolapsed uteruses and other weakened internal organs as it improves muscle tone. It also acts as a tonic for the genitourinary tract. It helps improve appetite and malabsorption problems and lessens lumbar pain and weak sensations in the legs and knees. False unicorn eases nausea and vomiting during pregnancy and in combination with other herbs helps to prevent miscarriages. It strengthens the spleen and raises overall energy in the body. When taking the root for its tonic qualities, drink 2–3 cups of tea a day or take 25–35 drops of tincture, two to three times a day, four to five times a week, for one to three months.

Note: Some old herbals say that nausea and vomiting can occur when large amounts of false unicorn root have been taken. I have never seen this happen. As with any herb, start out with small doses and gradually increase to recommended dose.

FEVERFEW (*Tanacetum parthenium*) *Asteraceae* or *Compositae*,
Daisy Family
Other common names: Featherfew, midsummer daisy, flirtwort,
featherfoil.
Parts used: Leaves and flowers.

Feverfew was brought to the United States by colonists from Europe, where it was widely used in traditional folk medicine. Feverfew is easy to cultivate in gardens. It is a perennial and once established will reseed itself freely. The roots will remain growing as a perennial if the flowers are pinched back as soon as they begin to form. Since I like to encourage them to reseed, I let some plants go to seed and I pinch others back. In Maine we start seeds indoors in late March and set the plants out into the garden in late May. Indoors, seed germination takes one to two weeks and the soil needs to be maintained at 70°F. Seeds need to be free of mold and not more than one year old to ensure good germination. Feverfew can also be propagated by dividing plants in the spring or fall.

Feverfew grows one to four feet high. It prefers fairly rich, loamy, and well-drained soil, and likes to be spaced twelve inches apart, either in a sunny location or in partial shade. Our plants respond well to adding compost into the bed and then mulching with compost or seaweed. The plant has lots of yellowish green leaves, one to three inches long, which are deeply and irregularly cut like chrysanthemum leaves. The small flowers have a flat yellow center with a single row of white ray flowers surrounding it. There are several cultivars available at greenhouses with different types of flowers. If you have ever eaten a fresh feverfew leaf you will most likely remember its distinctly bitter and camphory taste. After harvesting a few pounds of leaves, which I do just before the plant flowers, my fingers taste and smell of feverfew for several days.

I first began reading about feverfew as an herb for women after hearing one of my students speak of how effective the fresh leaf tincture was for helping ease her menstrual cramps and slow, sluggish menstrual flow. It is not uncommon for women with cold hands and feet to experience a delayed or sluggish menstrual flow. Taking feverfew for a few months, two times daily, four to five days a week, either as a fresh tincture, 25–50 drops, eating 1–3 fresh leaves, or taking a freeze-dried preparation, 50–100 mg per day, may help remedy this situation. Dandelion root and blessed thistle can be used with feverfew to improve liver health.

Feverfew's bitter components act as a digestive stimulant and liver decongestant. The action upon the liver improves sluggish menstrual flow and decreases feelings of pain and congestion in the pelvic area. Consider taking this herb before and after a D and C.

Feverfew helps to calm nerves and uplift the spirit. In some of the old herbals, including *A Modern Herbal*, by Mrs. M. Grieve, feverfew is said to be effective in "hysterical" complaints in women. Women's *hysteria*. I have often wondered what people really meant when they used this word. The root meaning of hysterical means "of the womb." Many of the old medical textbooks, both allopathic and herbal, use *hysteria* to describe a range of "women's problems" they say originate in the womb. No wonder removing the uterus is such a common practice today—a practice that needs serious thought given to its necessity.

Feverfew has received lots of acclaim recently for its proven effectiveness in treating migraine headaches of a vasoconstrictory type. Some research points to preventing migraine headaches by eating a few fresh leaves every day over several months or taking freeze-dried capsules. A tea or tincture of feverfew, dandelion root, and lavender flowers, taken one or two times a day, four or five times a week, for one to four months, along with a change of diet and adequate rest, may reduce and eliminate headaches and migraine headaches associated with the menstrual cycle. Feverfew is also being used on a daily basis by people with arthritis to reduce inflammation and pain. (Having an experienced homeopath take a person's history and prescribe a constitutional homeopathic remedy based on the individual's case has been helpful in eliminating migraine headaches for some people.)

For migraine and other chronic headaches: Take 15–25 drops of feverfew tincture, two times a day, or eat 1–3 fresh leaves daily for six months to a year. The consistent use of this herb over an extended period of time will allow you to see if the feverfew is working. Headaches, nausea, and vomiting will become less frequent and less severe over time if feverfew is effective for you.

Note: Avoid use during pregnancy. For people sensitive to strong oils, the fresh leaves may cause a skin irritation or mouth ulcers.

LADY'S MANTLE   (*Alchemilla vulgaris*) *Rosaceae*, Rose Family
Other common names: Lion's foot, bear's foot
Parts used: Leaves, flowers, and root

This cultivated perennial is native to western and central Europe and grows easily in well-drained soil. The grayish green leaves are soft, rounded with folds, three to eight inches in diameter, and resemble a cloak. The lacy flowers bloom in our gardens for two weeks in late June and look like a beautiful yellow cloud. The tap-root is black and fairly thick and the plant grows up to one-and-a-half feet high. In Europe there are over three hundred *Alchemilla* species, whereas in the United States *vulgaris* is the most widely grown.

Dew drops collect on the outer rim and in the center of the leaves and sparkle in the early morning sun. My friend Adele Dawson taught me to taste the dew from the leaves. I love to gently place my hands under the soft leaves and my face in the leaves, taste the fresh dew, and feel its

Lady's Mantle

wetness on my face. This has become one of my daily morning rituals in the garden. I'm sure the garden fairies get a good laugh watching me licking the leaves.

An easy way to establish this plant in a garden is from a root cutting. The mother plant sends out lots of side shoots that can be easily separated by cutting the roots with a spade or clippers and then transplanted. Plants grow in full sun or partial shade, tolerate slightly acidic soil, and are very winter hardy. The fuzzy leaves are some of the earliest to begin uncurling themselves in our gardens in April. Be sure when placing a lady's mantle plant into the ground that you dig a hole deep enough for the plant to sink into, and then stamp the soil firmly around the plant. This prevents the plant from heaving up during winter thaws. Lady's mantle will also reseed herself if you let some flowers go to seed. Keep your eyes open for baby plants and transplant them to an appropriate bed, or give some to your women friends.

The leaves and flowers are harvested when the flowers first begin to bloom. When making a tincture, I like to harvest the flowers and leaves at dawn when they are laden with dew. Wait until the dew is gone before collecting the plant for drying. Lay the leaves and flowers onto screens for drying, or hang the flowers in bunches from the ceiling to use later for dried flower arrangements.

Lady's mantle is a wonderful herb, more commonly revered by European than American women because of how prolifically she grows both in the wild and in gardens there. Many of my Dutch friends have at least two different species of *Alchemilla* growing in their tiny backyard gardens. Lady's mantle helps relieve mild aches and pains during the menstrual flow. The tea or tincture helps stop spotting between periods and lessens excessive menstrual bleeding for women of any age. Lady's mantle is also a supportive friend for women going through menopause. It eases physical and emotional discomforts. Lady's mantle's astringent nature is useful for diarrhea and as a mouthwash for sores. I have seen tinctures of lady's mantle and shepherd's purse used together topically as a wash or poultice help tighten and tone atrophied abdomen and forearm muscles and sagging breasts. A tea of lady's mantle and raspberry leaves taken daily for several weeks is helpful for a prolapsed uterus.

The moundlike way lady's mantle grows and its softness, reflect the beauty of women's bodies. She is an affirming plant to have growing near us. If all you have is a tiny space near your door for a few plants, do consider lady's mantle. She will bring joy and sparkle into your life for many years as she continues to grow fuller and rounder. If you have more room in a garden, find a special spot for several plants. Let this be a resting and healing place for you and other women to gather and be reminded of your beauty and women's wisdom.

MOTHERWORT   (*Leonurus cardiaca*) *Labiatae*, Mint Family
Other common names: Lion's tail
Parts used: Leaves and flowers

Different species of motherwort originated in Europe and Asia, and the European species, *Leonurus cardiaca*, has now naturalized in many places in the United States. You will often see her growing wild along the edges of fields and around old barns. She is easy to start from seed and reseeds herself freely in the garden. In

1986 I dug up thirteen wild plants from a nearby field and brought them to my gardens. Motherwort now appears throughout the garden wherever she wants, and often needs to be weeded out of certain beds. Her flower stalk grows from two to eight feet tall and creates a strong presence in the garden.

Motherwort flourishes in a well-drained, sandy soil that is slightly alkaline. I have observed her to grow taller when a bit of compost has been added. Motherwort is happiest when planted in the sun, but can grow in partial shade. The main stem is square, fairly thick, and has many leaves at the base that have three to seven unequal, toothed lobes. The upper leaves are lanceolate and deeply lobed, reminding me of fingers. The flowers are fuzzy and white or lightly pink with purple spots and can prick you with their sharp points. If you look at the flower with a hand lens you can see the upper lip of the flower has lots of hair on the backside. The pink lips of each flower look like the opening to a vagina, so common to flowers in the *labiatae* family. We harvest the leaves and the entire flower stalk with clippers when the flowers are in full bloom, anywhere from late June into August, being sure to leave enough flower stalks for reseeding to occur.

Tincture the leaves and flowers as soon as you pick them. If you prefer to dry them, lay the leaves and stalks onto screens. Motherwort tea has a very bitter taste. You may want to taste some tea before drying the plant. If you dislike the bitter tea, you can tincture the plants while they are still fresh.

The name *motherwort* indicates her useful qualities for many women's conditions. She helps bring on a delayed or suppressed menstrual flow, especially when someone is anxious and tense. Motherwort strengthens and relaxes the uterine muscles and eases uterine cramping. She is a mild heart tonic and aids in reducing rapid heartbeats brought on by nervous anxiety and heart palpitations during menopause. She is an ally for women during menopause as she helps relax and support the body through this changing time.

Motherwort eases early labor pains and calms the nerves after childbirth. Take motherwort only once soon after giving birth as consistent use before the uterus has clamped down may cause bleeding to continue. Use one to two times a day in the weeks following birth for easing tension and supporting a woman through the wide array of feelings that come with the newness of mothering.

Leonurus cardiaca means lion hearted. I think motherwort is strong medicine for women to put in dream pillows, to have in dried flower arrangements near our beds, by the telephone, in our workplaces, and to have growing in our gardens. We need courage to heal the various ways we have been wounded and have not been allowed to be the powerful, intelligent, wise women that we are. Motherwort gives us courage to be our true selves and to develop a strong heart, like the lion's heart. Strong hearts filled with courage are able to do anything. It takes a lot of courage to mother ourselves and children in a world that does not yet entirely value mothering, women, or children.

Motherwort mixed with lemon balm, linden flowers, raspberry leaves, blue vervain, fennel seed, borage flowers and leaves, and chamomile tea, relaxes and soothes the soul and brings happiness, strength of the trees, sweetness of the bees, and courage to those who partake of these herbs.

Note: Avoid using for menstrual cramps when bleeding is heavy. Also avoid during pregnancy.

WILD YAM   (*Dioscorea villosa*) *Dioscoreaceae,* Yam Family
Other common names: Rheumatism root, colic root
Part used: Root

This vining perennial plant grows wild in rich, moist woods from southern New England to Tennessee and westward to Texas. The leaves are heart shaped with hairs on the underside. The lower leaves grow in whorls of three to eight and alternate further up the vine. Wild yam is a favorite plant of mine to spot while walking in the woods because of its viney nature and obvious leaf veins. The roots are spiny and very tough to cut. Several autumns ago, while collecting wild yam roots, I was gifted with a root that grew in a circle instead of straight. I saved this root and it now sits upon the altar in my medicine-making room.

Native American women used wild yam roots in a tea to ease labor pains and today we are fortunate to have information about this plant from native women. Wild yam root is effective in relieving ovarian pain and uterine cramps before and during menstruation. I often use wild yam in combination with other herbs to regulate a woman's menstrual cycle, to bring on menstrual bleeding that has been absent for several months, to lessen premenstrual stress, and to ease hormonal changes and hot flashes during menopause.

Wild yam works well in combination with crampbark and false unicorn root to prevent miscarriage (see formula listed in chapter 7). It is useful to use for promoting fertility and normalizing hormone production after a miscarriage or abortion. It is also effective for nausea and vomiting during pregnancy.

Wild yam is an excellent remedy for relieving intestinal gas and muscular spasms of the intestines and for healing various liver and gallbladder problems. It is a liver-tonic herb I often consider using when the hormonal system and liver both appear to be in need of support. It is safe for long-term use. Wild yam eases intestinal colic and is an herb to consider for diverticulitis. It reduces the acute inflammation of rheumatoid arthritis and eases joint stiffness when taken two to three times a day over several months.

YARROW *(Achillea millefolium)*
  Compositae, Daisy Family
  Other common names: Milfoil
  Parts used: Flowers and leaves

White yarrow grows abundantly in the fields that surround my gardens, in the western foothills of Maine where I grew up, and on many islands off the coast of Maine. Every now and then I will come upon a lightly colored pink flower in my wanderings, which I do not pick because they are not that common here. Over eighty species of *Achillea* are found in various parts of the world. Some common cultivars seen in perennial gardens in the United States are the Golden Yarrow, *Achillea filipendulina*, and the Rose Yarrow, *Achillea millefolium roseum*, a pink-to-magenta colored yar-

Yarrow

row. These cultivars are not to be picked for tea or tincture, only for pleasure and for fresh and dried flower arrangements.

I feel a special affinity for the wild yarrow because it has a reputation for having been used by the village herbalists of Europe along with the elder flowers. For me this plant embodies memories and wisdom that were lost during the witch-burning times. Even though herbal information disappeared as herbalists were killed, many plants survived and still contain the knowledge that women are tapping into today by gardening, wildcrafting, and using herbs.

The leaves of yarrow are beautiful, finely dissected and feathery, growing two to eight inches long, becoming smaller near the flowers. This soft and distinctively fragrant perennial grows one to three feet high. Each tiny flowerhead has five petal-like ray flowers, one-quarter inch wide and the entire flower cluster is three to four inches wide.

Yarrow can be propagated by seeds or root divisions in the spring or fall. Space the plants ten to twelve inches apart as they will spread. Yarrow does much better growing in full sun and in slightly acidic soil (pH 4.5–7). I transplanted lots of yarrow clumps from a field area I was about to rototill and cover crop. They transplanted easily. Every three or four years I divide yarrow clumps to stimulate growth.

I gather the flowers as they first open and tincture some immediately, laying the rest on screens to dry for tea and for special herb bundles. Yarrow tea, or tincture, is useful for easing menstrual cramps. Chamomile and catnip are useful additions to your teapot alongside the yarrow for relieving mild cramps and for relaxing the body. Yarrow helps to bring on a delayed menstrual cycle and because of its astringent nature can be used to lessen a heavy menstrual flow.

Yarrow in combination with elder flowers, catnip, and peppermint is a favorite old-time remedy among many herbalists for bringing down a fever when it's taken as a hot tea. Yarrow and boneset are also two herbs I commonly use together during a cold or flu. Because of yarrow's bitter taste it is a good digestive stimulant when taken as a cool tea. Because of its astringent qualities it can be used for diarrhea and dysentery, and can be applied topically to allay bleeding and help heal wounds. A yarrow poultice or salve helps stop bleeding from hemorrhoids and aids in their healing.

I include yarrow in herb bundles for protection while traveling and in a pouch for someone who is asking to reconnect with the green world. White yarrow made into a flower essence is beneficial for anyone who is easily depleted by external influences and absorbs negativity. In *The Flower Essence Repertory*, the Flower Essence Society writes

> Those who typically need this remedy are easily affected by their surroundings, and can be prone to many forms of environmental illness, allergies, or various psychosomatic diseases. Such persons have an extraordinary capacity for healing, counseling, or teaching, because they are readily able to receive psychic information and to understand the pain and suffering of others. At the same time they are easily depleted, and are quite vulnerable to the thoughts or negative intentions of others. Yarrow quite literally "knits together" the overly porous aura of such an individual so that it does not "bleed" so excessively into its envronment. . . . Yarrow bestows to the Self a shining shield of Light which protects and unifies the essential Self, allowing compassionate healing qualities to flow freely from one's soul to others.[11]

You may want to consider planting yarrow near your house or at the entrance to an herb garden. This plant radiates beauty and light.

HERBAL FORMULAS

FIRST MENSTRUAL BLOOD

Each woman's menstrual story is unique and influenced by things like cultural and family customs, sexuality issues, economics, and religion. Future generations of young women will grow up feeling freer in their bodies and easier about menstruation as more women today acknowledge and claim their female wisdom, power, and right to choose which kind of sexual relationships they wish to have, whether they be lesbian, bisexual, or heterosexual. I believe that as some kind of positive recognition of this major female transition is reintroduced into Western culture, fewer health problems related to our female organs will occur. Honoring this passage into womanhood connects a young woman with the natural flow of life in her body and to an experience that belongs fully to women. Welcoming a young woman into the community of women in whatever way feels okay to her helps break the isolation, fear, and shame that many women feel about their bodies.

Young Woman's Tea

The following herb blend is a nourishing and tonic tea for young women to drink when they first begin bleeding. To experience full tonic effect, drink one to three cups daily, four to five times a week over several months, deleting the mugwort after the first month.

Red raspberry leaves—2 parts

Lemon balm—2 parts

Lavender flowers—1 part

Sweet marjoram—1 part

Alfalfa leaves—1 part

Nettle leaves—1 part

Mugwort flowers and leaves—1 part

Dose and Use: Pour 1 cup of hot, steaming water over 2–3 teaspoons of herbs; steep, covered, five to ten minutes. Strain and drink 1–3 cups per day. Or place 4–6 tablespoons of herbs into a glass quart jar, fill jar with boiled water, cover, and steep five to fifteen minutes.

The liver support herbs listed in chapter 5 can be helpful to take four to five times a week in addition to the above tea.

Red Fruit Delight

Mix strawberries and raspberries together with a touch of maple syrup and garnish with fresh borage or heartsease pansy flowers in summer, or mix with yogurt and maple syrup. Bake a favorite lemon cake and pour the following fruit syrup on top.

Heat 1 cup of apple cider or juice. Dissolve 1 heaping teaspoon of kuzu (available at food co-ops and health food stores) in ⅓ cup of cool water and slowly add to hot juice, continuously stirring so no lumps form. Add 3–4 tablespoons of maple syrup, a squirt of lemon juice, and place as many fresh or frozen strawberries and raspberries as you want on top of the cake and pour the hot fruit syrup over the fruit.

Yoni Tea

This tea mixture is an all-purpose women's tea. The mineral-rich herbs strengthen and tone the reproductive organs, ease menstrual cramps, and stimulate an overall feeling of well-being. They are safe and nourishing for pregnant and nursing women to drink on a daily basis. Consider drinking this tea several times a week, even if you are not pregnant, for its health-promoting properties.

Red raspberry leaves—2 parts

Alfalfa—1 part

Nettle leaf—1 part

Red clover—2 parts

Peppermint—1–2 parts

Dose and Use: Pour 1 cup of hot steaming water over 2–3 teaspoons of dried herbs and steep, covered, five to ten minutes. Drink warm or cool. For sipping throughout the day, place 4–6 tablespoons of herbs in a glass quart jar and fill with hot water, secure cover, and let steep five to ten minutes, or longer if you prefer a stronger tea. This tea can be made into a sun or moon tea. (Directions for these teas is in chapter 2.)

BUTTERFLY KISSES

Accidentally, this morning
while stretching in bed
my arm feels the familiar
yet strange thrill—
the brush of dry insect wings.
Where did I first learn,
forgotten, remembered, forgotten again,
of the finer uses of eyelashes
Must have been a group of us girls
sharing our secrets and laughing
around our first blood-time.

—Nancy Devine

Hormonal Balancing Formula

The following herbs are helpful from the onset of menstruation through menopause. This particular combination strengthens and tones the reproductive organs, brings hormones back into balance after coming off the pill; after an abortion or miscarriage; after a long illness or an extended use of drugs, including antibiotics; or after surgery, i.e., removal of ovarian cysts or fibroids, or a cesarean. Helpful for regulating the menstrual cycle and reducing menstrual cramps when taken over several months. Take with Yoni tea. Use after giving birth to tone the reproductive organs.

Blessed thistle leaves and flowers—1 part

Dong Quai root—1 part

False unicorn root—2 parts

Licorice root—½ part

Vitex berries—3 parts

Dose and Use: Take as tea or tincture. For most effective results, take over many months, two to three times per day, four to five times a week. Tincture: 15–30 drops each time. Tea: drink 2–3 cups per day. To make tea, simmer the roots, covered, for twenty minutes. Add in leaves and flowers and steep, covered, for ten to twenty minutes. Take this combination throughout the month for several months until you feel the balancing changes these herbs offer. Cease taking this formula if you become pregnant or during your menstrual flow. If cramping occurs, use herbs listed under menstrual cramps.

Premenstrual Support Herbs

The following herbs support the hormonal changes that occur one to two weeks before menstruation begins. When these herbs are taken over a period of time—two to six months—they assist in relieving nervous anxiety, mood swings, irritability, swollen and sore breasts, water retention, and cramping.

Chasteberries—3 parts

Crampbark—2 parts

Motherwort—2 parts

Oatstraw—1 part

Sarsaparilla root—2 parts

Dose and Use: Take two to four times per day from ovulation through bleeding. As a tincture, take 15–40 drops. To make tea, pour 1 cup of hot steaming water over 2–3 teaspoons of herbs and drink 2–4 cups a day. If cramping occurs before bleeding, add your favorite herbs for relieving menstrual cramps. If you experience discomfort all month, take this formula throughout the month. Diet, exercise, acupuncture, homeopathy, and emotional support are other factors that can help improve your overall health.

Herbs for Easing Menstrual Cramps

The following herbs help ease menstrual cramps before and during menstruation.

Crampbark—2 parts

Black cohosh root—2 parts

Wild yam root—2 parts

Ginger root—1 part

Rose petals—1 part

Dose and Use: Take as tincture, 15–40 drops in water or tea, three to six times per day or 10–30 drops every half hour. For severe cramps take 20–40 drops of valerian root tincture with the above herbs. Pulsatilla tincture can be helpful for women who feel weepy generally or who burst into tears easily before and during their menstrual flow, and skullcap helps to ease tension and emotional anxiety. Add 10–15 drops of either or both herbs when needed to above formula.

Moon Tea

The following tea is soothing and relaxing. Give yourself a few moments to sit down and sip a cup of tea when you first begin to bleed. Drink 2–4 cups a day. Alternate with Yoni tea for variety. Add a touch of mugwort or southernwood to call in the energy of Artemis.

Red raspberry leaves—2 parts

Lemon balm—2 parts

Lemon verbena—2 parts

Oatstraw—1 part

Lavender—1 part

Lady's mantle flowers and leaves—½ part

Sweet marjoram—1 part

Rose petals—½ part

Dose and Use: Pour 1 cup of hot steaming water over 2–3 teaspoons of herbs and steep, covered, five to ten minutes. To make a quart to sip throughout the day, put 4–6 tablespoons of herbs in a glass quart jar, fill with hot steaming water, cover, and let steep five minutes or longer.

Amenorrhea Remedy

Amenorrhea is the absence of menstruation. Each woman's situation is different and must be taken into account when designing a formula. Some possible causes of amenorrhea include excessive exercising, traveling, stress, coming off the pill, weight gain or loss; other causes can be emotional blockages, anemia, or anorexia nervosa. It is important to use herbs that help regulate the hormonal system, support

the reproductive organs, and have emmenagogue properties along with addressing any emotional issues.

The following herbs help bring energy to the pelvic
area, increase blood circulation throughout the body, redi-
rect blood flow to the pelvic area, and regulate hormonal
function.

Wild yam root—2 parts

Blue cohosh root—1 part

Vitex berries—2 parts

Dong Quai root—1 part

Mugwort flowers and leaves—1 part

Ginger root—1 part

Dose and Use: Take in tincture form, 25–50 drops, three to
four times per day, for a minimum of three months. Continue taking for three months even after bleeding begins to
ensure the hormonal system is balanced and strong. After
using for three months, reevaluate your changes and adjust
the formula according to your needs. If you have not bled
for many months or years, the guidance of an experienced
herbalist, Chinese practitioner, acupuncturist, or homeopath may be useful to you.

Drink Yoni tea, Moon tea, and your favorite nervine herbs.
Have a moon party and invite other women friends to bring red
food, flowers, and inspiring images to help you visualize your blood
flowing again.

Emmenagogues Herbs

If your menstrual flow is late and you know you are not
pregnant, the following herbs can help stimulate the menstrual flow. Many kinds of stresses–cold, tension, shock,
emotional upsets, traveling, and school, work, or family
pressures–can cause a period to be late.

Freshly grated ginger root tea increases circulation to the pelvic area and helps bring on a late menstrual flow, especially if the pelvic area feels cold or congested. Drink hot, 4–6 cups per day. Grate 1–2 tablespoons of fresh roots and simmer in one cup of water, covered, for ten minutes. Add lemon and honey if you want. Soaking your feet for ten to fifteen minutes in hot ginger tea also improves circulation to the pelvic area. Adding 1–2 drops of the essential oil of ginger and pennyroyal to a 1-ounce bottle of mugwort oil (made with a vegetable oil) and massaging the feet and belly also increases circulation and feels relaxing.

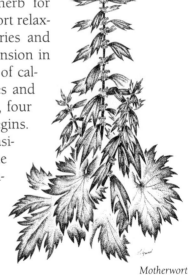

Motherwort is my favorite herb for bringing on a late period. Motherwort relaxes the nervous system, eases worries and fears, and releases tightness and tension in the body. You can add equal parts of calendula flowers and mugwort leaves and flowers and take as tea or tincture, four to six times a day, until bleeding begins. The tea is bitter tasting and often easier to take in tincture form. Get in the bathtub if you have one, light a candle, add a few drops of the essential oils of mugwort and melissa, and dream of bleeding.

Motherwort

Herbs for Menorrhagia—Heavy Menstrual Bleeding

Heavy bleeding with the menstrual cycle can be caused by fibroids; an infection; a hormonal imbalance, especially as a woman approaches menopause; vascular congestion; excessive intake of aspirin, caffeine, salt, red meat, estrogen, and drugs. As you investigate the root cause be sure to replenish your body with nourishing and iron-rich foods, good quality protein, and plenty of rest. Floradix is an excellent liquid herbal iron supplement available through food co-ops and health food stores to restore iron and so is taking nettle and yellow dock root tea or tincture three times a day for several weeks or months.

The hormonal balancing formula and Yoni tea and liver-tonic herbs such as dandelion, burdock, and wild yam root can be taken four to five times a week over several weeks or months to support the endocrine system and liver. Use the following formula to help lessen heavy bleeding during your menstrual flow.

Shepherd's purse—2 parts

Lady's mantle leaves and flowers—2 parts

Yarrow—3 parts

Partridgeberry leaves—1 part

Dose and Use: Take 20–60 drops of tincture four to six times a day when bleeding, or take 30–50 drops every hour or more if needed.

Anemia Formulas

The following two formulas were created by herbalist Matty Becker. The first is specific for heavier-built women or women who consider themselves to be overweight. The herbs improve the body's ability to absorb nutrients by strengthening the body's natural eliminative channels, promoting healthy blood cells, and assuring that the food eaten is transformed into usable nutrients. (The herbs that have an asterisk after them are Chinese herbs. Refer to the herb resource list for mail-order sources.) The yellow dock syrup described in chapter 5 is a simple and effective remedy to take over several weeks for anemia if you do not wish to use Chinese herbs. Floradix, an herbal preparation available in health food stores, is also useful for anemia.

Astragalus root*—2 parts
Yellow dock root—1 part
Dandelion root—1 part
Burdock root—1 part
Nettle leaves—1 part
Hu shu wu*—1 part

Dose and Use: Simmer 6 tablespoons of roots in one quart of water for one hour and then add the nettles and steep for one hour. You can also simmer the roots for twenty to thirty minutes, add the nettles, and steep for eight hours. Take ¼–½ cup, three times per day before eating for as many weeks as you feel necessary. Use for at least one month. Store tea in refrigerator for up to three days.

This formula is for women who are thin, may be run down and undernourished, and are vegetarians; or for women who are not able to eat enough nutrient-rich food. This formula also gives strength and nourishment to women who are challenged with anorexia nervosa.

Dong Quai*—1 part
Cooked rehmannia*—1 part
Saw palmetto berries—1 part
Codonopsis root*—1 part
Hu shu wu*—1 part
Jujube dates*—½ part

Dose and Use: Simmer 6 tablespoons of herbs for one hour in 1 quart of water, or simmer twenty to thirty minutes and then steep for eight hours. Take ¼–½ cup, three times per day before eating for at least two months, or longer if needed. Store tea in the refrigerator for up to three days.

Migraine Headache Relief

Some women experience migraine headaches in association with their menstrual cycle. Hormonal changes, emotional stresses, food and environmental allergies, caffeine, misaligned vertebrae, and oral contraceptives may be some of the possible causes of migraines. Some avenues to explore in reducing and eliminating migraines include: acupuncture; homeopathy; diet changes, which include avoiding dairy and cold foods and reducing intake of sugar, fruit, caffeine, and alcohol; liver-toning and hormonal-balancing herbs taken over several months; and body work to realign the spine and improve posture. Be as kind and patient with yourself as possible. Migraines usually take a few months or even longer to decrease in severity.

The following herbs help to ease a migraine headache. Take as tea or tincture whenever you feel a migraine or regular headache coming on.

Feverfew—3 parts

Lemon balm—1 part

Passion flower—½ part

Rosemary—1 part

Sacred basil—1 part

Ginkgo leaf freeze-dried capsules or tincture—2 parts

Dose and Use: Pour 1 quart of hot, steaming water over 6 tablespoons of herbs and steep, covered, five to fifteen minutes. Drink ½ cup every hour until symptoms subside. The herbs can be taken as a tincture, four to six times a day, 30–60 drops.

Add a few drops of the essential oils of lavender, marjoram, or lemon balm to a warm bath and ask a friend to massage your head, neck, and feet.

MOON GARDEN

If you garden, you may want to create a moon garden with special plants to sit near when you bleed. Let yourself visualize shapes, colors, textures, and smells that are pleasing to you and make a special area to sit near or lie in. Some of the flowers and herbs I especially love are red tulips, bleeding hearts, red bee balms, poppies, yarrow, fragrant lilies, irises, sweet-scented carnations, pink cosmos, and rosemary.

In the past year I have been creating a crescent-shaped moon garden with plants that have silvery foliage or white flowers. Some of these plants include a white flowering butterfly bush, white delphiniums, campanulas, dianthus, lamb's ears, lavender, veronica, speedwell, Russian sage, garden sage, sweet alyssum, baby's breath, white foxglove, phlox, nicotiana, cosmos, clary sage, British silver mullein, English daisy, snow in summer, and cleomes.

I have a particular fondness for the Greek goddess Artemis and cultivate various plants of the genus *Artemisia* in her honor, some of which grow in my moon garden. The pre-Hellenic Greek myths viewed Artemis as the protector of children, animals, and women giving birth. She roamed freely through the woods and fields and was wise in the uses of medicinal plants. Artemis loved whomever she chose and was owned by no one. Some plants whose genus is *Artemisia* include: mugwort (*Artemisia vulgaris*), French tarragon (*Artemisia dracunculus sativa*), southernwood (*Artemisia abrotanum*), wormwood (*Artemisia absinthium*), roman wormwood (*Artemisia pontica*), sweet Annie (*Artemisia annua*), silver queen (*Artemisia nutans*), silver king (*Artemisia ludoviciana albula*), and silver mound (*Artemisia schmidtiana*).

Many herbs have stories associated with them. You may want to grow certain herbs for strengthening and supporting specific areas in your life. For example, rosemary is considered to be the herb of remembrance, helping a person remember dreams and the ancient wisdom deep within. Thyme offers people courage and support in speaking out. Mugwort, also called cronewort, is the bringer of dreams. Any of these herbs in dried form are a nice addition to a dream pillow, special pouch, anointing oil, or herb bundle for burning as incense.

Moon Garden

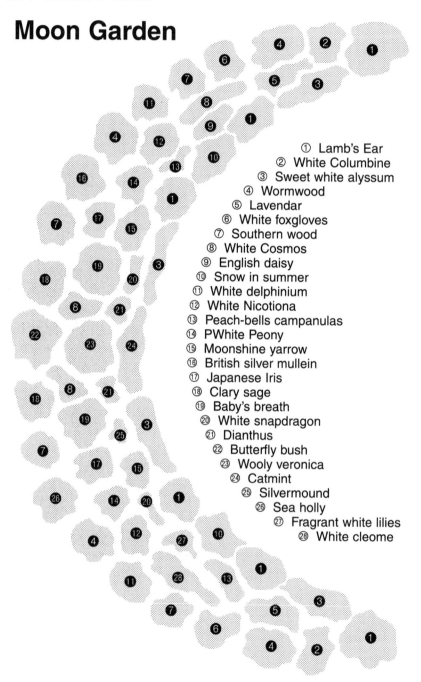

① Lamb's Ear
② White Columbine
③ Sweet white alyssum
④ Wormwood
⑤ Lavendar
⑥ White foxgloves
⑦ Southern wood
⑧ White Cosmos
⑨ English daisy
⑩ Snow in summer
⑪ White delphinium
⑫ White Nicotiona
⑬ Peach-bells campanulas
⑭ PWhite Peony
⑮ Moonshine yarrow
⑯ British silver mullein
⑰ Japanese Iris
⑱ Clary sage
⑲ Baby's breath
⑳ White snapdragon
㉑ Dianthus
㉒ Butterfly bush
㉓ Wooly veronica
㉔ Catmint
㉕ Silvermound
㉖ Sea holly
㉗ Fragrant white lilies
㉘ White cleome

7

Pregnancy and Birth

We know ourselves to be made from this earth. We know this earth is made from our bodies. For we see ourselves. And we are nature. We are nature seeing nature.

—SUSAN GRIFFIN

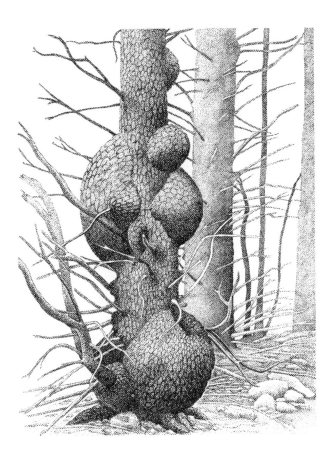

Mothering ourselves and children is a multifaceted job. Many mothers tell me it is the most wonderful and the most difficult thing they have ever done. In Western countries, mothering is not regarded as central to a community's well-being, even though the message women receive when girls is that to be a "real woman" is to have children. Society assumes that women know how to be mothers just because we live in a female body. This is an extremely hurtful assumption for women who are unable to become pregnant, for women who do not become mothers, for women who choose to have an abortion, for women who experience a C-section, or when mothering becomes challenging. The whole subject of pregnancy and parenting for lesbians is another challenging issue rarely supported or openly discussed among women, health care providers, or society at large.

The following information comes from the many women I have worked with over the past twelve years. Included are herbs that support a woman recovering from a C-section. Several photographs of babies who came into this world with help from herbs now hang in Avena's lab. These babies and their moms are living testimonies to how effective herbs are. Though I am not a trained midwife, I have assisted at many births and have great respect for the tradition midwives are carrying on. To mother children is one of the most important tasks any person can do.

Fertility Herbs

Every woman's body, health needs, and story is unique and varied and comes into play when she tries to become pregnant. The following herbs offer support and nourishment to the hormonal system, uterus, and liver.

Dong Quai root—1 part

False unicorn root—1 part

Vitex berries—1 part

Blessed thistle leaves and flowers—½ part

Dose and Use: Simmer 6 tablespoons of the roots and berries in 1 quart of water for fifteen minutes and add 1–2 teaspoons of blessed thistle, steep, covered, five to fifteen minutes. Drink 2–3 cups per day, four to five times a week. Alternate with Yoni tea. As a tincture, take 25–50 drops, three times a day, four to five times a week.

When you are ovulating, light candles and speak to your ancestors. Ask for help in being open to receiving new life.

Discontinue the herbs, except Yoni tea, when you become pregnant. Yoni tea is described in chapter 6.

MISCARRIAGE PREVENTATIVES

The following tincture and tea are helpful to use throughout the first trimester of pregnancy if you have a history of miscarriage or are spotting early on in your pregnancy.

Tincture

False unicorn root—1 part

Wild yam root—1 part

Crampbark or black haw root bark—2 parts

Dose and Use: Take 25–50 drops of tincture, two to four times per day as a preventative, or every two hours until spotting stops. Consult your midwife or doctor for support and information, especially if bleeding continues.

❀

Tea

Raspberry leaves—1 part

Oatstraw—1 part

Lemon balm—2 parts

Nettle—1 part

Partridgeberry leaves—2
parts

Dose and Use: Place 6 tablespoons of herbs in a glass
quart jar and fill jar with hot
steaming water. Steep, covered, ten to fifteen minutes
and drink throughout the
day for several weeks along
with taking above tincture.

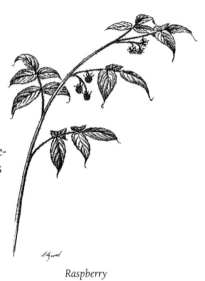

Raspberry

TERMINATING A PREGNANCY

The issue of using herbs for terminating an unwanted pregnancy is
a big one. Women around the planet have always known which
herbs to use. There are pockets of women who still have these
skills, though this information is harder to find in Western cultures.
The following books offer personal and compassionate insights and
alternative information for women looking for support: *Self-Ritual
for Invoking Release of Spirit Life in the Womb* by Deborah Maia and
A Difficult Decision: A Compassionate Book About Abortion by Joy
Gardner.

MISCARRIAGE OR POSTABORTION SUPPORT

Experiencing a miscarriage or abortion brings up lots of emotions.
Support from friends and/or family is essential at this time, along
with the help herbs, flower essences, homeopathic remedies, body
work, acupuncture, counseling, and other therapies offer.

If you are miscarrying, have a close friend with you for support, especially in helping you stay present in your body and aware of your body's process. The Bach flower essence called Rescue Remedy, available at most health food stores, can help calm your emotional state. If you have a midwife she may also offer homeopathic or herbal support.

If you have a scheduled clinical abortion, take arnica homeopathic pills, 30c, two times a day, the day before, the day of, and one to two days following to ease the shock and trauma of this experience. Rescue Remedy can also be taken as often as needed. Have your partner or a close woman friend with you for emotional support. Many women have found that creating some kind of releasing ritual, either before and/or after gives them permission to grieve and allows their emotional healing to be more complete. Be gentle—grieving takes time.

The following herbs help to support the hormonal system, remove blood clots that may be left, move stagnant blood, and revitalize and renew the blood following a miscarriage or abortion.

False unicorn root—1 part

Vitex berries—1 part

Motherwort—1 part

Wild oats—1 part

Dong Quai—2 parts

Dandelion root—1 part

Dose and Use: Take as tincture, 25–35 drops, three times per day, for one to two months. Drink 1–3 cups of Yoni tea daily for several months along with your favorite nerve tonic herbs.

PREGNANCY, LABOR, AND BIRTH SUPPORT

Herbs to Avoid During Pregnancy		
Barberry root bark	Poke root	Pennyroyal
Mugwort	Thuja	Rue
Southernwood	Senna	Tansy
Wormwood	Cascara sagrada	Goldenseal
Feverfew	Juniper berries	

Nausea With Pregnancy

There are many reasons for women feeling nausea in the early stages of pregnancy or even throughout the entire nine months. The hormones are shifting quickly because the body suddenly finds itself pregnant. Low blood-sugar levels and the body's need for more nutrition are areas to address in helping remedy this situation.

The following herbs support the liver and hormonal system. Consult with a midwife or doctor about good quality prenatal vitamins.

Wild yam root—2 parts

Meadowsweet—1 part

Dandelion root—1 part

Peach leaves—1 part

Fennel seed—1 part

Dose and Use: Easiest to take in tincture form, 25–40 drops, three to four times day. During acute times, take 10 drops as often as needed. Eat easily digested foods that appeal to you—some ideas include yogurt, miso vegetable soups, barley and slippery elm bark gruels with a touch of ginger, tamari, or miso, crackers, and kuzu gravies added to cooked brown rice.

Drink 3–4 cups of Yoni tea, warm or cool, each day. Add a touch of herb honey; sacred basil is my favorite. Other safe and nourishing herbs to combine in different ways with raspberry could include lemon balm, oatstraw, linden blossoms, and sweet marjoram. Warm ginger root tea can also be helpful in easing nausea.

Exhaustion

Some women feel exhausted in the early months of pregnancy. Remember you are now eating for two beings. Do your best to eat nourishing foods and rest. Dandelion root and leaves, yellow dock root and leaves, and nettle leaves can be taken as a tea or tincture two to three times a day if you feel tired and run down. They increase iron and help your body better assimilate nutrients. Floradix, a commercially prepared herbal liquid, is also an excellent remedy for low iron. Yellow dock syrup with black-strap molasses is a good remedy too (listed in chapter 5). Refer to foods listed under iron in chapter 6.

SONOGRAM AND AMNIOCENTESIS SUPPORT

Be well informed and clear about why you are doing either of these two procedures. Take Rescue Remedy as often as you need before and after to help ease any anxiety or fear you may feel. Have your partner or a good friend along for emotional support. Talk to your baby before, during, and after the procedure to let her or him know what is going on and why. Medical procedures such as sonograms and amniocentesis disrupt the flow of energy in the body. You may want to have some body work after the procedure like polarity, reiki, or shiatsu to help rebalance your body's energy flow. Flower essences can also help rebalance the body's energy.

LABOR SUPPORT

The following herbal suggestions come from my own experiences of being a support person at several births, some at home and some in hospitals.

Flower Teas

Birth can be a very special, powerful, and magical time for the woman giving birth and for her helpers. Wherever you choose to give birth, surround yourself ahead of time with beautiful things like flowers, stones, seashells, drawings, or other items that offer you support and remind you of your connection to Earth and other women. Drinking a tea of any of the following herbs serves to uplift your spirit, gladden your heart, and nourish your nervous system. It is particularly useful when you are in a hospital or any other sterile environment; after giving birth, or whenever you feel overwhelmed, depressed, or disconnected from yourself and nature. I call this mixture Fairy Flower Formula.

Sacred basil leaves and flowers—2 parts

Lemon balm—2 parts

Borage flowers—1 part

Lavender flowers—2 parts

Heartease pansy flowers—1 part

Dose and Use: As a tincture, take 5–10 drops as needed. Continue to drink as much raspberry-leaf tea or Yoni tea throughout labor or chew ice cubes made from raspberry tea.

Other Herbal Aids for Birthing

The red oil made from fresh St. Johnswort flowers is a must to have at all births. I hope someday it will be available in all birthing centers and hospitals. This oil is very soothing to rub on the perineum during labor and especially valuable after birth has occurred. The oil is anti-inflammatory, eases any swelling and burning pains, and heals tears very quickly. Keep it near the toilet with your squirt bottle of water and put it on the perineum every time after you urinate. Use for as many weeks as you need.

Motherwort, skullcap, and lavender can be used every hour as a tea or tincture to help calm and relax the body during labor. Rescue Remedy can be placed on a woman's head, on her lips, in her tea, or under her tongue as often as needed throughout labor to help calm her and allay anxiety, stress, or fear. Have these herbs mixed ahead of time either in tincture form or ready for a friend to make into tea.

Two herbs I like to place near a woman during birth are rosemary and mugwort. Rosemary is the herb of remembrance and helps a laboring woman remember that every woman who has ever given birth is with her, supporting her as she gives birth. Rosemary is also nice to have near the baby to help the baby remember her/his connection to the spirit world as she/he is born. Have a plant in the birthing room, keep a bundle of dried rosemary stalks near, burn rosemary, place rosemary essential oil in a diffuser to add fragrance to the room, or place the essential oil of rosemary on your wrists to smell during labor.

Mugwort is the herb associated with the goddess Artemis, protector of women during childbirth. Have a bundle of dried mugwort near to remind you to call upon Artemis to help you as you labor. You can burn mugwort oil and rosemary together. Have someone massage you with mugwort oil or place the oil on your forehead and wrists. If you want to take a bath in the early stages of labor, add mugwort and rosemary tea or the essential oils to your bathwater and let yourself rest in the arms of Artemis.

Mugwort

If complications occur during labor and delivery, be sure to have your support team give you Rescue Remedy and place drops on the baby once she/he is born. If the baby is whisked away, place Rescue Remedy on the baby as soon as you are reunited. A student of mine gave birth eight weeks early a few years ago, and her daughter was placed in an incubator for several weeks. My friend would drop Rescue Remedy and cauliflower flower essence on her fingers and then touch her baby through the small opening every day when she visited her.

Arnica homeopathic pills, 30c and 200c, are excellent to have in your birthing kit to give after labor for healing bruising of the vagina or labia; if the mother feels shocky, is exhausted and shaky, has trauma to the soft tissues because of a big baby; if suction is used to pull out the baby; to help prevent postpartum bleeding; and to use for mother and babe if the birth was long and difficult. If you feel bruised and sore after having a vaginal birth, take arnica homeopathically, soon after giving birth and every two to three hours until the pain ceases.

Take arnica before and after a C-section to ease the trauma and shock of surgery. If you have a planned C-section, begin taking arnica, 30c, the day before your surgery, three times a day.

A homeopathic consultation for the baby and mother can be

beneficial after any kind of birth trauma to help release the trauma and prevent future health problems.

Postpartum Bleeding

Fresh shepherd's purse tincture, 40–60 drops, given in water soon after birthing, acts quickly to stop bleeding because of its hemostatic and vasoconstricting properties. Repeat again every two to five minutes if needed. Twenty to 30 drops of blue cohosh tincture can be given once along with shepherd's purse to help the uterus clamp down. Some midwives give 15 drops of blue cohosh and 15 drops of shepherd's purse tinctures in raspberry tea after the baby is born and before the placenta is delivered. Continue giving shepherd's purse tincture if needed. Continue giving raspberry leaf tea.

Postpartum Support

The liver needs herbs to support the rapid hormonal changes that occur after the body is no longer pregnant and to help in eliminating any drugs that were given.

The following liver-support herbs are valuable for any woman who has given birth. They are especially important for a woman who has experienced a C-section, was given a spinal anesthetic, Pitocin, or any other drugs. Little nourishing and rebuilding support is offered to women in the hospital after experiencing a vaginal birth or C-section. Many women have grueling headaches for a few weeks after a C-section and are commonly told to drink coffee. Coffee weakens the liver and is irritating to a woman in such a vulnerable state as well as unhealthy for her newborn baby.

> Blessed thistle—1 part
> Bupleurum root—3 parts
> Dandelion root—2 parts
> Wild yam root—1 part
> Astragalus root—1 part

Dose and Use: Take as a tincture, 25 drops, three to four times per day, after meals, for one to two months. Bupleurum is a commonly used Chinese herb for releasing stuck energy in the liver. This is an important herb to use after a C-section because the liver meridian is severed during this procedure.

Surgery weakens and depletes the body of nutrients. Be sure to eat nourishing foods high in iron, protein, and minerals after a C-section. Have your friends take turns bringing food into the hospital. Continue drinking Yoni tea and/or a mother's nursing tea.

A good quality Siberian ginseng root tincture helps rebuild the immune system, increases the white blood cell count after surgery, reduces the toxic effects of drugs, and, when taken consistently over two to six months, increases energy and stamina. Take 15–25 drops, three times per day for two to six months after giving birth.

Herbal Sitz Bath

Make a strong infusion by pouring 1 quart of hot steaming water over 6 tablespoons of comfrey leaves. If you have calendula and yarrow flowers add 2–3 teaspoons of each of them into your quart jar and steep thirty minutes or longer. Strain the herbs and add the tea into your warm-water sitz bath tub. Other things that help to speed up healing perineum tears include resting (movement aggravates tears), direct exposure to sunlight, and taking 400 IU of Vitamin E, twice daily, and Vitamin C, 2000–4000 mg daily.

Herbs to Ease Postpartum Pain and Nervousness

The following herbs can be taken soon after birth and during the month following to ease afterpains and anxiety and nourish and calm the nervous system.

Black cohosh roots—2 parts

Crampbark—2 parts

Wild yam root—1 part

Motherwort—1 part

Hops—1 part

Dose and Use: Take as a tincture, 15–30 drops, three to five times a day.

Postpartum Tonic

The following herbs help bring hormone levels back to balance, tone the uterus, nourish the nervous system, and uplift the spirit. Some postpartum headaches or feelings of depression can be caused by a hormonal overload, lack of oxygen to the brain, or liver congestion. Daily use of these herbs eliminates these headaches.

Blessed thistle—1 part

Vitex berries—2 parts

Dong Quai root—1 part

False unicorn root—2 parts

St. Johnswort—1 part

Sacred basil—1 part

Dose and Use: As a tincture, take 25–50 drops, three to four times a day for two to four weeks. As a tea, simmer 3–6 tablespoons of the roots and berries, covered, in 1 quart of water. Take off the heat, add in 2–3 tablespoons of the leaves and flowers, and steep, covered, another five to fifteen minutes.

Postpartum Tea for Relaxing

Lavender flowers—1 part
Chamomile flowers—1 part
Catnip—1 part
Lemon balm or lemon verbena—2 parts
Lady's mantle—1 part

Dose and Use: Place 6 tablespoons of herbs into a glass quart jar and fill the jar with hot steaming water. Cover and steep five to ten minutes, strain, and drink warm or cool throughout the day, with or without honey.

Postpartum Anemia and Exhaustion Remedy

The following Chinese herbs make an excellent nutritive tea to drink two to three times a day for three to four weeks after giving birth to replenish iron, rebuild the blood, and increase energy and strength.

Cooked rehmannia—2–3 parts
Dong Quai roots—1–2 parts
Codonopsis root—1 part
Astragalus root—1 part
Ho shu wu—2 parts
Jujube dates—1 part

Dose and Use: Place 12 tablespoons of the herbs in 2 quarts of cool water, let sit overnight, and then simmer for one hour. Drink 1–3 cups a day for one to three months. Store extra tea in refrigerator up to two days.

Nursing Mother's Herbal Tea

The following herbs are rich in minerals and vitamins and stimulate healthy milk production.

Red raspberry leaves—2 parts

Nettle leaves—1 part

Borage leaves—1 part

Blessed thistle leaves and flowers—
1 part

Fennel seed—3 parts

Dose and Use: Place 4–6 tablespoons of herbs in a glass quart jar and fill with hot steaming water. Steep, covered, for five to ten minutes, or longer if you like strong tea. Drink 1–4 cups a day.

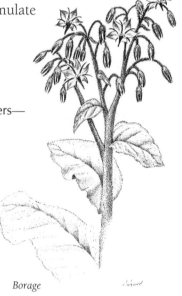

Borage

Newborn's First Bath

Any combination of catnip, chamomile, lavender, rose petals, and lemon balm is wonderful to place in the first bathwater. The herbs are gentle, kind, soothing, and calming. Place 6 tablespoons of herbs in a glass quart jar and fill with hot steaming water. Steep, covered, for ten to fifteen minutes. Strain and pour the warm tea into the bathwater. A few fresh flowers floating in the bathwater add a special touch for mother and babe.

8

Stories Our Vaginas Tell

As a woman, I feel the answers for our inner balance come to us from our relationship to the Moon, the Earth, our relationship with the feminine and masculine energy within us, and our ancient memory as "green women," healers of the Earth. . . . In this day of scientific research and of dependency and orientation on allopathic medicine, many of us have lost faith in the power of ceremony and prayer for healing and maintaining good health. . . . By reclaiming our heritage as healers, by loving the Earth and listening to her teachings, and by caring for ourselves with loving compassion, and with the use of gentle, natural remedies, we create the balance that brings well-being and vitality in all its fullness.

—ROSEMARY GLADSTAR

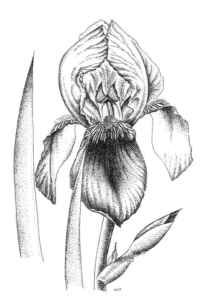

*T*his chapter contains explanations and herbal formulas for women's health conditions that have some connection to the vagina. The herbal remedies listed are suggestions to help you choose what is best for your unique situation. Some of the herbs may be effective for you, and others may not. Work with the herbs that you feel an affinity to and ones that are accessible to you. Seek appropriate medical care when needed.

Using herbs gives you the opportunity to participate in your healing process. Become more familiar with your particular health situation and the herbs you decide to take. Fear and confusion can arise when working with certain conditions such as condyloma (genital warts) or herpes. Many of us were taught to quickly ingest medicine and go on to something else, hoping whatever is "wrong" will disappear. Pause for a moment before taking herbs or allopathic drugs. Take a deep breath and visualize your body healing. Ask the medicine to assist your body's healing process. The healing energy of the Earth and Universe is here to support you.

DIETARY AND NUTRITIONAL CONSIDERATIONS

A nourishing and well-balanced diet is an important place to begin strengthening and healing our bodies. The quality, quantity, and manner in which we take in food all play a major role in our overall health. Our systems and organs are all interconnected and an imbalance in a certain area can lead to problems in other areas. The internal ecology of the vagina is a reflection of the whole body's health.

A simple diet, low in fats, sugars, and processed foods and high in whole grains, beans, nuts and seeds, dark leafy green vegetables, root and sea vegetables, and other foods appropriate to your climate, culture, and bioregion strengthens the body. (Refer to resource section for cookbooks.)

Vaginal Infections (Vaginitis)

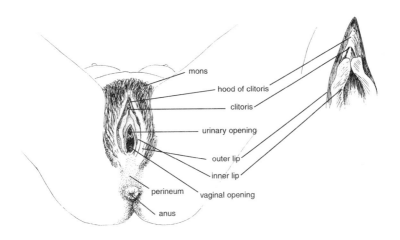

The vagina is part of our whole body. Often the conditions that precipitate an infection are rooted in the circumstances of one's life. Infections have a tendency to occur when your resistance has been lowered by things such as exhaustion, emotional and mental stress (including disturbing or abusive childhood memories surfacing), drugs, antibiotics, douches, birth control pills, hormone replacement therapies, vaginal sprays, alkaline and deodorized soaps, tampons, frequent or abrasive intercourse, lack of sleep, and high intake of sugar and fruit, caffeine, or alcohol. If your resistance is lowered you are more susceptible to getting certain vaginal infections from a sexual partner who has an infection.

Some women are plagued by chronic vaginal infections even after following guidelines for reducing them. Infections that persist after using prescription drugs can be frustrating and demoralizing. Women with long-term, recurring infections often receive their best emotional support from women with similar circumstances. It is not always easy to be patient and nurturing to ourselves when we feel agitated, uncomfortable, and discouraged. Finding a safe and loving environment to talk about your feelings, family history, and past traumatic experiences can open doors for deeper healing.

At different points during the monthly cycle, the mucus from the vaginal membranes may be white, clear, slippery, yellow, thick, or thin. These normal secretions do not cause the vulva or vagina to become inflamed. Many kinds of bacteria grow in the vagina. Lactobacillus is the most prevalent one, and it keeps the vagina's pH level slightly acidic. The vagina's pH level is normally around 4.0 to 5.0. This acidity level ensures that an overgrowth of yeast, fungi, protozoa, and bacteria does not occur. When any of these organisms multiply and upset the ecological balance of the vagina, they irritate the vaginal walls and cause infections. This results in abnormal discharges of various colors, smells, and consistencies; mild or painful itching; a burning sensation; and sometimes frequent urination. Usually changes in hygiene, diet, and living habits reduce or eliminate a mild vaginal infection.

Note: Recurring vaginitis can be a symptom of a serious underlying problem such as a sexually transmitted disease, chronic cervicitis, or an ascending infection of the genital tract. Find an open-minded and compassionate family doctor or obstetrician/ gynecologist, nurse practitioner, physician's assistant, or naturopathic doctor who can guide you.

Prevention of Vaginitis

- Wear clean cotton underwear and avoid underclothes, including pantyhose, made from nylon or other synthetic material. Synthetic fibers do not breathe and therefore retain heat and moisture that foster the growth of harmful bacterias.
- Avoid wearing tight pants. The friction causes the vaginal membranes to become inflamed.
- Wash your vulva with your hands and pat yourself dry. Washcloths breed germs. Washing your vulva with your hands also gets you in touch with your body. Many of us were reprimanded for touching and exploring our vaginas as young girls.
- Use soap sparingly and avoid daily use. Alkaline soaps diminish the acidity of the vagina and destroy the body's natural oils, which protect us from infections. Avoid all vaginal sprays, as they disrupt the vaginal flora. (Where did the

notion that women's vaginas smell bad come from? How come sprays for men's penises aren't mass-marketed?)

- Avoid talcum powders. Recent studies show that they may cause ovarian cancer.[1]
- Avoid douching whenever it's possible to use another treatment. Douching destroys the friendly bacteria that produce the protective acidity of the vagina.
- Decrease caffeine, chocolate, sodas, alcohol, sugars (including honey), and sweetened and unsweetened fruit juices. Diets high in sugar change the vagina's pH.
- Make sure your sexual partner(s) is clean and keeps her or his nails short. The risk of getting an infection from a woman lover is far less than for a woman with a male lover. (Few studies on lesbian health have been done and there is a great need for more specific information on how lesbians pass infections to each other.) Various infections can be passed to a woman from a male lover. The regular use of condoms is advised since it adds protection against many kinds of infections, including HPV (human papilloma virus). HPV-caused lesions found on the cervix put a woman more at risk for cervical cancer. An abnormal Pap smear can indicate if HPV is present and a colposcopy is often used to find warts or flat lesions. A biopsy is usually recommended to diagnose HPV if lesions are found. If either partner has a genital infection, avoid intercourse until it is cleared up.

SUPPLEMENTS

The following recommendations are useful for any form of vaginitis.

Vitamin C–1000–3000 mg, two to three times daily up to bowel tolerance.

Beta-carotene–50,000–75,000 IU, twice daily with meals.

Vitamin E–400 IU daily with food.

Zinc–15 mg daily with food. (Picolinate is its most absorbable form. Avoid prolonged use of zinc if taken without copper as you can develop a relative copper deficiency.)

Organic flax-seed oil–2–3 teaspoons, twice daily mixed with grains, vegetables, or soup.

Lactobacillus bifidus powder (type of acidophilus)–use a good quality from a health food store. Keep stored in refrigerator. Take ½ teaspoon twice daily, between meals. Follow directions on bottle.

Yeast Infections (Also called candida, monilia, or fungus)

Yeast–*Candida albicans* or *monilia*–is a one-celled plant that normally lives in the vagina. Yeast organisms and lactobacillus (a bacteria) both live and feed on the sugar (glycogen) from vaginal secretions and from cells that are sloughed off during the menstrual cycle. Yeast infections occur when the pH of the vaginal environment changes.

Antibiotics, high-sugar diets, and prolonged periods of stress are three common factors that cause the vagina's pH to change and yeast to multiply. The vagina's pH level increases just before and during menstruation, allowing yeast to flourish, which is one reason why some women experience small amounts of itching around their labia at this time. The pH level rises when oral contraceptives, hormone pills, antibiotics, and other drugs are taken. Candida is common in pregnant women because of heightened pH levels due to hormonal changes.

For women having intercourse with men, semen raises the vagina's pH for several hours following contact. Also, some women having intercourse develop yeast infections because men can carry candida under their foreskins, though men rarely develop yeast infections themselves. It is rare but Candida can be transmitted between women by oral sex, if the "oral" partner has thrush, a yeast infection of the mouth.[2] When yeast is budding in the vagina, it is best to avoid putting any objects, tampons, or fingers into the vagina, since any disturbance of these buds will spread the yeast organisms.

Symptoms of Yeast Infections

- Mild to intense itching, irritation, and redness of vagina and vulva.
- White, curdy discharge that smells yeasty or sweetish. Usual odor of the vagina is pleasant and musky.

- Patches of white discharge on the vaginal walls and cervix that may be seen with the aid of a speculum.
- Frequent urination accompanied by a burning sensation occurs for some women.

To ensure that the infection is yeast, a small sample of discharge can placed on a microscope slide in saline or 10 percent potassium hydroxide and examined for the buds or branching hyphae, characteristic of yeast that are actively reproducing.

Herbal Support Formula

The following herbs are effective for clearing up candida and other fungal and yeast overgrowths in the vagina as well as in the urinary tract, mouth, and on skin and nails. These particular herbs are most effective when used in tincture form. To avoid the alcohol present in a tincture, boil a small amount of water, place drops in water, and let alcohol evaporate before drinking.

Echinacea purpurea roots—2 parts

Black walnut hulls—2 parts

Usnea—3 parts

Spilanthes leaves and flowers—2 parts

Goldenseal root—1 part

Dose and Use: 30–60 drops, mixed in a small amount of water, and taken orally, three to six times per day.

Ti Tree Oil

Herbalist Hart Brent recommends that her clients with persistent candida infections place 2–3 drops of a good quality ti tree oil into a ½ teaspoon of honey and take orally, twice a day, for three days. Take a break for four days and repeat the following week if needed.

Yogurt

Yogurt with active cultures (homemade when possible) can be used by soaking a tampon in yogurt with 2–3 drops of ti tree oil and inserting into the vagina at night. (Decrease number of drops or eliminate ti tree oil if membranes feel more irritated.) The live lactobacillus culture found in freshly made yogurt helps eliminate a yeast infection by repopulating the gastrointestinal tract and balancing vaginal yeast growth. Use for six consecutive nights. Break for two nights and repeat if needed.

Acidophilus Capsules

Acidophilus capsules can be used instead of yogurt to restore normal flora. Insert two acidophilus capsules per night, for five to six consecutive nights. Break for two nights and repeat if needed.

Garlic

Peeled and un-nicked garlic can be wrapped into unbleached gauze with a string attached and placed inside the vagina overnight for up to six consecutive nights to eliminate infection.

Eating fresh garlic daily also helps clear up yeast and bacterial infections. Garlic is antifungal, antibacterial, and antiviral. Add fresh garlic to soups and vegetable stir-fries after they are done cooking. Garlic is an excellent food source for keeping the body healthy and for preventing infections, particularly in these times when we are faced with air and water pollution and other environmental toxins. Fresh garlic becomes easier to eat over time.

Ti Tree Oil Suppositories

I have seen wonderful healing results for women with chronic yeast infections with ti tree oil suppositories. These suppositories are available through the mail from Wise Woman Herbals (see resource list). If you are unable to obtain a good quality ti tree oil suppository, you can buy "00" size gelatin capsules from the drugstore and with a dropper place 1–2 drops of ti tree oil into the capsule and fill the rest of the capsule with usnea or calendula oil. For women who wish to avoid using gelatin, an animal by-product, ask at a health food store for an alternative. Insert 2 capsules nightly for six consecutive nights.

Herbal Douche

Dilute 1 tablespoon (5 ml) of ti tree oil into 2 cups (500 ml) of warm water. Add 2 tablespoons of apple cider vinegar. Fill a plastic disposable douche bottle (available for $2–$3 at drugstores) with this solution. Follow directions on the package. Be very gentle when squeezing the bottle. Douche two times a week, allowing two to three days between each douche. Use acidophilus capsules or the yogurt tampon the other nights until symptoms are gone.

Boric Acid Capsules

Some holistic and even some allopathic health care providers suggest using boric acid powder, available from most pharmacies, for eliminating persistent yeast infections. Add a tiny pinch of slippery elm bark powder into each "00" size gelatin capsule and fill with boric acid powder, not crystals. Insert 2 capsules into the vagina at night for one week. Apply an herb salve to the labia to help prevent a burning sensation. As the capsule dissolves internally there will be some "mild" burning in the vagina for the first few days. If the burning continues beyond the first few days, stop using the capsules. You will want to sleep on a towel and use a pad during the day because some vaginal discharge will occur. After completing a week with the boric acid capsules, insert either acidophilus capsules or yogurt-soaked tampons for one week to restore normal flora along with taking an acidophilus supplement orally.

Caution: Do not ingest the capsules. They are poisonous. Be sure to keep them away from children and animals.

Plantain

Ripe plantain seeds can be gathered from the seed stalks in late summer, dried, and stored in a jar. Soak them in a small amount of boiled water. The seeds will form a gel. This gelatinous liquid can be gently placed onto inflamed labia to help reduce itching and swelling and heal open sores. Plantain leaves, fresh or dried, can be made into an infusion for rinsing sore and inflamed areas, or included in an herb salve.

Digestive Herbs

The following herbs nourish and rebuild the digestive tract and liver. They are helpful to take in conjunction with the above herbal support formula if you experience chronic yeast infections. To receive the most benefit, use two to three times per day, for four to six weeks. Then cut back to one or two times daily, three to four times per week and continue for another few months if needed. If you have complications or suspect a serious digestive, liver, or kidney problem, seek appropriate medical help.

Digestive Aid

Dandelion root—2 parts
Burdock root—1 part
Gentian root—2 parts
Licorice root—1 part
Blessed thistle leaf—2 parts
Nettle leaf—1 part

Dose and Use: If you are using the above herbs as tea, take 4–6 tablespoons of roots and simmer in a quart of water, covered, for twenty to thirty minutes. Take off the heat and add 2 teaspoons each of blessed thistle and nettle. Let steep ten minutes, covered. Drink 2–3 cups per day, twenty minutes before eating. To use tincture, place 25–50 drops in a small amount of water that has just boiled. Let sit five minutes and take orally.

Irritated Vulva

If your vulva or labia itch, are swollen, irritated, and red, rinse affected or infected areas with a strong tea made from calendula and chamomile flowers, and chickweed and comfrey leaves as often as you want. You can apply an herb salve made in a vegetable oil (avoid petroleum-based salves) with calendula, St. Johnswort flowers, and plantain and chickweed leaves. Yogurt can also be applied to the external genitalia to soothe and help replenish normal flora. There is no need for women to suffer and not know the simple herbs that bring relief and healing.

TRICHOMONAS

Trichomonas vaginalis is caused by a one-celled protozoan called a trichomonad. It is a parasite that is present in the vagina, intestines—including the rectum of many women and men—and in the urethra of many men. It can be transmitted through contact with wet objects like towels, underwear, swimsuits, and washcloths; wiping oneself from the rectum to the vagina; by exchanging vaginal secretions between women if one woman has a trichomonas infection; through sexual intercourse; and through anal contact followed by vaginal contact without proper washing in between during sexual interactions. Trichomonas multiplies when the vagina's pH level is raised by similar kinds of stresses discussed under yeast infections.

Trichomonas is most often passed on by sexual contact and both sexual partners will need to be checked. If your partner is a woman, and either of you have trichomonas, avoid exchanging vaginal secretions until the infection is cleared up. Rest when you can, take naps together, and be creative in sharing sexually. If your sexual partner is a man and he is diagnosed with trichomonas, he can soak and wash his penis in a dilution of the herb tinctures suggested below, two to four times per day, along with taking the herb tincture orally, also two to four times per day. Avoid sexual intercourse until the infection is cleared up. Support each other's healing in whatever ways you can.

Symptoms of Trichomonas

- Red, tender vulva.
- A thin, foamy or frothy vaginal discharge that is yellowish green in color and unpleasant smelling, sometimes described as having a dirty-sneaker smell.

- Itching, swelling, or bleeding of the vaginal walls or vulva.
- Burning pain upon urination. Burning sensation can mean other things also.
- Red, strawberry spots on the cervix or vaginal walls.

Dietary and Herbal Support

Follow the same vitamin and dietary guidelines for a yeast infection along with supporting the overall health of the immune system. I have seen the herb usnea work well for eliminating trichomonas infections. Usnea can be made into a tincture and taken orally or diluted with warm water for douching and made into an oil or salve for topical application.

❀

Immune Support Tincture

Usnea—4 parts
Echinacea root—2 parts
Licorice root—1 part
Calendula—1 part
Thuja—1 part
Goldenseal root—2 parts

Dose and Use: Take 25–50 drops of tincture mixed with a small amount of water orally, two to three times per day, five to six days a week, until the infection is cleared up. Drink lots of oatstraw, calendula, and nettle tea for added nourishment.

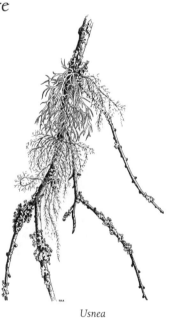

Usnea

Vaginal Suppositories

Use the ti tree oil suppositories listed under yeast infections. Many naturopathic doctors have seen good results with ti tree oil suppositories.

Vaginal Douche

Use the douche listed above under yeast infections if you cannot obtain ti tree oil suppositories.

Standard Medical Treatment

Flagyl (metronidazole) is the usual medical treatment for trichomonas. There are many possible side effects with the use of flagyl, including nausea, dizziness, cramps, yeast infections, diarrhea, joint pain, and numbness of arms and legs. FLAGYL IS UNSAFE FOR PREGNANT AND NURSING WOMEN AND WOMEN WITH CENTRAL NERVOUS SYSTEM DISORDERS, BLOOD DISEASES, AND PEPTIC ULCERS. AVOID INTAKE OF ALCOHOL IF USING FLAGYL.

Betadyne suppositories are milder than Flagyl and can be tried before using Flagyl. If you choose to use Flagyl, ask to take the single oral dose instead of the three- to seven-day treatment.

Note: If you take Flagyl be sure to support your body with a whole foods diet, the suggested supplements, plenty of rest, and clean water. Take a good form of acidophilus powder, orally, for several weeks along with drinking 2–3 cups of oatstraw, calendula, and nettle tea daily. Take echinacea root and usnea tincture, two to three times per day for the two weeks following Flagyl, then take three to four times a week for another month along with the Digestive Aid formula listed above. If your immune system is run down, follow guidelines listed in chapter 11. If you feel another infection coming on, immediately start taking the Immune Support Tincture listed above, four to six times per day along with following dietary and lifestyle recommendations. Seek appropriate medical care when needed.

BACTERIAL VAGINOSIS (FORMERLY CALLED GARDNERELLA OR HEMOPHILUS)

A combination of the various bacteria now called bacterial vaginosis (BV) is a common cause of vaginitis. Lots of women have an overgrowth of these bacteria and are asymptomatic. A fairly common way women who are asymptomatic discover they have bacterial vaginosis is when they have a Pap smear and the practitioner takes a swab of vaginal discharge and looks at it under a microscope. Mostly what is seen are cells, called clue cells, which have changed because of an overabundance of certain bacteria.

The main etiologic agent in BV is an increase in anaerobes in the vagina. The reason this occurs is unknown. Organisms commonly found include *Bacteroides*, *Peptococcus*, and a newly described bacterium, *Mobiluncus sp.* The last named organism is a small, crescent-shaped motile bacterium. These organisms may be accompanied by *Gardnerella vaginalis*, but *Gardnerella* can be found in 40 percent of women without BV. There is a decrease in the normal lactobacilli of the vagina but it is not known whether this is a cause or effect of the disease. Vaginal pH is increased in BV. The organisms present in BV cause the level of vaginal amines to be high. These amines are volatilized when the pH is increased, causing a characteristic odor.[3]

BV may be transmitted between women by exchanging vaginal secretions and between women and men through sexual intercourse. Proper hygiene is important as there is the possibility of transmission from wet towels and washcloths. However, recent medical research is showing some controversy as to whether BV is a sexually transmitted disease or whether BV occurs when the pH of the vagina is upset. Stress, high intake of sugar, and a poor diet are some things that upset the vaginal pH and set the stage for an overgrowth of bacteria.

Bacterial vaginosis is self-sustaining and becomes part of the stable flora of the vagina once it is established, making it much more difficult to disrupt. Over time BV can irritate the cervix and alter vaginal mucous membrane integrity.[3]

If a woman's cervix looks pink and healthy and there is no excessive vaginal discharge and the Pap smear reports no inflammation yet does report bacteria, she should not be concerned. If her cervix looks inflamed, or the Pap smear reports inflammation along with BV, then the problem should be addressed, even if she has no symptoms. A chronically inflamed cervix is more susceptible to the human papillama virus if exposed and the accuracy of a Pap is lowered when the cervix is inflammed.

Symptoms of Bacterial Vaginosis

- Heavy, thick, white, yellow, or gray discharge that usually smells unpleasant, sometimes fishlike.
- Burning with urination.
- Burning sensation in vagina after intercourse.
- Strong vaginal odor after intercourse.

Treatment for Bacterial Vaginosis

BV can be very stubborn. When designing a treatment plan, some important areas to consider include restoring the vaginal flora and stimulating vaginal mucousal immunity. Look for underlying explanations of why the vaginal flora is upset and support the immune system systemically. Herbal suppositories, herbal tinctures and teas, and a homeopathic constitutional treatment can all be helpful.

Dietary Support

Follow the same dietary and supplement guidelines previously listed.

Herbal Support for BV

Usnea—2 parts
Echinacea root—2 parts
Calendula—2 parts
Licorice root—1 part

Thyme—1 part

Ocotillo bark or leaf (optional)—1 part

Dose and Use: Take ½–1 teaspoon tincture orally three to five times per day. If you can tolerate the taste of chaparral tincture add 5–10 drops from a separate bottle into the water you are about to drink, which has drops from the above mixture. (I've found liquid rice dream, available in health food stores, to be a helpful liquid to add terrible tasting tincture drops to.)

Take a lomatium and goldenseal glycerite (available through some herb companies) for two weeks to help stimulate an immunological response in your body along with the herbal tincture listed above for BV.

Drink a tea made from calendula flowers, nettles, oatstraw, and plantain leaves along with liver-tonic herbs.

Drinking 8 ounces of unsweetened cranberry juice mixed with water daily helps to acidify your system.

Herbal Douche

Usnea—3 parts

Spilanthes—3 parts

Calendula—2 parts

Echinacea root—1 part

Oregon grape root—2 parts

Myrrh—1 part

Dose and Use: Place 50–75 drops of the above tincture into a quarter cup of hot, steaming distilled water. Let cool and mix with a quarter cup of calendula tea. Pour into a plastic disposable douche bottle, and gently douche for six consecutive nights. Use the herbal suppositories listed below, the following week (after douching) for six consecutive nights. Repeat this program for one month alternating douching and using the suppositories.

Herbal Suppositories

Alternate ti tree oil suppositories and usnea suppositories with acidophilus capsules nightly for several weeks. You can also use a calendula, Vitamin A, and echinacea vaginal suppository to help soothe irritated mucous membranes as needed. (See resources for suppliers of vaginal suppositories.)

Oxyquinaline Sulfate

Dissolve 2–6 oxyquinaline sulfate tablets (see mail-order resources) into warm calendula tea that contains ⅛ teaspoon of ti tree oil, place into a disposable plastic douche bottle (available for $2–$3 at drugstores), and very gently rinse your vagina without going up beyond the cervix. Do twice weekly for two to four weeks. Insert 2 acidophilus capsules nightly, five nights a week, for several weeks to help reestablish lactic acid in the vagina along with orally taking a good quality lactobacillus powder, twice daily, over several weeks or months if needed. Eliminating BV takes time.

To help relieve itching, rinse labia with a strong infusion of calendula, chickweed, plantain, and comfrey several times a day. Apply an herb salve directly onto the labia and inside the vagina with some of the same herbs, along with goldenseal and echinacea, as often as needed.

Be sure not to further aggravate or irritate the vaginal lining by having sexual intercourse or by inserting sex toys or other items into the vagina.

Standard Medical Treatment

BV is usually treated with antibiotics such as Flagyl (metronidazole) and tetracycline, sulfa creams, or suppositories.

CAUTION: Women of African and Mediterranean ancestry should be aware of possible side effects to sulfa drugs and probenecid. Pregnant women should never ingest Flagyl or tetracycline.[4]

Allopathic medicine may frustrate, embarrass, and discourage many women with chronic vaginitis, often making them feel dependent on drugs. It is important that women receive good information on how to replenish, rebuild, and nourish the body when taking drugs and also information on how to continue making dietary and lifestyle changes that support, heal, and prevent further infections. Often symptoms keep recurring because the underlying stresses are still present. Give yourself some quiet moments to rest and reflect upon your life when you can. Seek out appropriate medical support as needed.

VULVITIS

Vulvitis is an inflammation of the vulva and can be caused by various kinds of irritations from soaps, deodorants, synthetic underwear, sanitary pads, a decrease in hormone levels, or from rough or abusive touching. The vulva can easily become inflamed with any vaginal infection or herpes.

Poor eating habits and stress make women more vulnerable to vulvitis. Postmenopausal women are susceptible to developing vulvitis because, as their hormone levels drop, the vulvar tissues become thinner and dryer. Women with diabetes are also more susceptable because of higher levels of sugar in their vaginal cells, which causes higher vaginal pH levels.

SYMPTOMS

- Redness, soreness, itching, and swelling of vulva.
- Fluid-filled blisters can form and break open, releasing pus, and then crust over. A secondary infection can occur if these sores continue to be irritated.[5]

A vegetable-based oil or salve made with St. Johnswort, calendula flowers, comfrey root and leaves, chickweed, red clover, plantain, and goldenseal root, can bring down the inflammation, ease the pain and itching, and heal sores. Apply as often as needed. If the vulva is oozing pus, an herbal rinse made with any of the above herbs will help to relieve the discomfort. Rinse as often as needed.

HERPES

There are over five hundred types of herpes viruses, herpes simplex virus (HSV) being the most common among humans. Herpes simplex I causes the common cold sore around the mouth and herpes simplex II usually causes sores in the genital area. There can be some crossover if oral-genital sex is practiced. Herpes is transmitted during vaginal, oral, or anal sex with someone who has an active infection. Herpes spreads when the skin is red, and until the crusted-over scabs have disappeared. It also is transmitted when a person is asymptomatic. Herpes becomes incorporated into the DNA of the cells once someone is infected.

Usually symptoms begin to appear two to ten days after exposure, but the virus can remain dormant for several months or years. Genital herpes begins with an itching sensation in the genital area, which can last for a few hours or many days before the sores appear. Blisters appear on the outer and inner labia, clitoris, perineum, vaginal opening, and sometimes on the vaginal wall, thighs, anus, or buttocks. Blisters erupt within a few days and may ooze pus or blood. Some women experience pain, tingling, or a burning feeling in their legs and genital area. Painful and frequent urination, a vaginal discharge, and vulvitis can occur. The first outbreak is usually the most painful. Swelling of the lymph nodes in the groin, fever, and headache may occur.

Seventy-five percent of infected people experience a second outbreak of herpes within twelve months of their first flare-up.[6] A weakened immune system, an illness, menstruation, pregnancy, and traveling are all situations that can bring on a herpes outbreak. A deficiency in B-vitamins, an unbalanced diet, lack of sleep, and the use of birth control pills or antibiotics can increase the likelihood of an outbreak.

There is no allopathic "cure" for herpes. Fortunately, the frequency of flare-ups can be decreased with immune-strengthening herbs, diet, exercise, rest, and by reducing stresses. Reducing stress means different things for different people. Economic, social, and cultural factors influence the circumstances of a person's life and ability to reduce stress.

There is a 60–70 percent chance of a baby being born with a herpes infection, which can cause brain damage or death, if the mother has active sores and delivers vaginally. Find an experienced homeopathic practitioner or another holistic practitioner for guidance with natural remedies and diet along with consulting your midwife or doctor. I have seen several people with herpes drastically reduce their herpes outbreaks when on a constitutional homeopathic remedy.

Dietary Support

Avoid foods high in arginine on a long-term basis as they stimulate herpes: chocolate, cola, peanut butter, peanuts, cashews, pecans, almonds, sunflower and sesame seeds, peas, corn, coconut, and gelatin. Also keep your intake of sugar, fried foods, and white flour to a minimum.

Include foods in your diet with high lysine content: brewer's yeast, organic potatoes, and fish, if you eat fish. Eat lots of dark green leafy vegetables, whole grains, and garlic. Add a few teaspoons or more of kelp to your food every day. Blue-green algae is very expensive but can be helpful–3000 mg daily. A few teaspoons of organic flax-seed oil added daily to vegetables or rice has a nice buttery flavor and strengthens the immune system. Eat as much raw garlic as you can. Add garlic at the end of preparing soup or steamed vegetables.

Supplements

The following supplements are recommended for long-term use unless otherwise specified.

Lysine–1000 mg, two to three times per day for three months

Beta-carotene–25,000–50,000 IU, twice daily with meals

Vitamin C–1000–2000 mg, two to three times daily, up to bowel tolerance

Vitamin E–400 IU, daily with meals

Zinc—15 mg daily

A good B-complex vitamin

Note: Pregnant women are advised to discuss supplement doses with their health care provider.

HERBS FOR GENITAL SORES

Warm sitz baths with strong infusions of calendula flowers, comfrey leaves, plantain, and chickweed soothe and heal open sores. Prepare 2–4 quarts of the tea and add to a sitz bath. Soak at least twenty minutes. Let your vulva air dry after a bath. The sores often heal faster when exposed to air. Wear cotton underwear and avoid tight clothing. Apply an herb oil or salve only after vulva is dry and has had some exposure to air each day.

A whole-body bath with a few quarts of a strong infusion of calendula, oatstraw, linden, and comfrey added along with a few drops of lemon balm essential oil is very calming and relaxing.

An oil or salve made with calendula and fresh lemon balm and St. Johnswort flowers heals sores around the mouth and in the genital area. Apply as often as needed. Calendula is antiseptic and helps reduce swelling and pain, heals open sores, and prevents scarring. St. Johnswort flowers are anti-inflammatory, reduce pain and a burning sensation, and heal open sores. A drop of the pure essential oil of lemon balm can be applied topically along with the salve as lemon balm is antiviral. Salves also heal sores after crusts have formed.

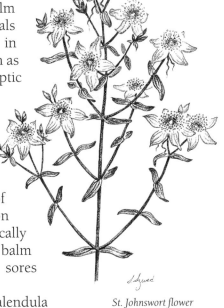

St. Johnswort flower

A tincture of fresh calendula flowers, fresh lemon balm, licorice root, or propolis can be carefully applied onto an open lesion with a piece of cotton or the end of a Q-Tip. The alcohol will sting at first, but effectively dries up lesions.

A paste made with equal parts of slippery elm bark powder, goldenseal powder, and echinacea root powder moistened with calendula or licorice root tincture and applied directly onto the sores brings symptomatic relief to painful sores. Apply salve or oil after carefully cleaning the paste off your skin. Dry goldenseal powder can be applied directly onto open sores to facilitate healing. Some people find the juice from an aloe vera plant to be soothing and healing to the sores.

A commercially prepared product for health care providers made with red Alaskan dulse and peppermint oil by Sozo Natural Products has proven to be very effective at eliminating pain and facilitating a quick clearing of the herpes lesion for some naturopathic doctors.

Use a plastic squirt bottle to spray water over genital area when urinating if the urine burns your sores. Let yourself air dry before putting your clothes on.

Herbs for Internal Use

The following herbal formula supports and nourishes the immune system and nervous system. Take it if you feel herpes symptoms coming on or are in a stressful situation that could stimulate an outbreak.

Echinacea root—1 part

Spilanthes—1 part

Calendula flowers—2 parts

St. Johnswort flowers—2 parts

Licorice root—1 part

Siberian ginseng root—1 part

Dose and Use: As a tincture, place 25–50 drops in water and drink three to four times a day, for two weeks. If symptoms persist and/or you still feel tired and run down, continue using these herbs one to three times a day, four to five days per week, over several months. Rebuilding your immune system helps prevent the frequency of herpes outbreaks.

Nervous System Tea

The following herbs strengthen the nervous system. Drink 2–4 cups daily when you feel stressed, vulnerable, if you know you will be in a stressful situation, during a herpes outbreak, or whenever you want.

Oatstraw—2 parts

Nettle—1 part

Calendula—1 part

Lemon balm—2 parts

Skullcap—1 part

Linden—2 parts

Dose and Use: Place 6 tablespoons of herbs into a glass quart jar and pour boiling water over the herbs, secure the lid tightly, and let steep ten to twenty minutes. Drink throughout the day, warm or cool.

CERVICAL INTRAEPITHELIAL NEOPLASIA
(CERVICAL DYSPLASIA)

Cervical intraepithelial neoplasia (CIN) is the scientific term for the abnormal development of cells on or near the cervix. It is usually diagnosed by a routine Pap smear. Different classification systems are used to determine how much of the surface tissue of the cervix is affected by abnormal cells and to what degree the cells have changed.[7]

It is hard to tell exactly where a woman is in the classification system. Be sure to get a second Pap smear and discuss various treatment plans with your health care provider before making any decisions. Abnormal cells (class II) often return to normal, though some women with CIN find their abnormal cells progress rapidly into cancerous cells. Doctors usually recommend more frequent Pap smears or other diagnostic techniques to monitor abnormal cell changes. Find a holistically minded doctor to work with and, if possible, a naturopathic doctor experienced with CIN and natural treatments.

Risk Factors for CIN

- If you or your sexual partner has had many sexual partners.
- Human papilloma virus infections are linked to an increased risk of cervical cancer. If you are sexually active with a man, find out if he has HPV, because the virus is passed during intercourse if the partner is infected. HPV is less often transmitted between women partners though still possible.
- Herpes simplex II is being linked to cervical cancer.
- Teenage women who have intercourse are at higher risk because the cells in the vagina are still changing during these years. The softer cells, which have not yet been replaced by tougher, squamoculumnar cells, are more vulnerable to whatever causes abnormal cell growth.
- Exposure to carcinogenic substances in the home or workplace.
- Long-term use of oral contraceptives.
- Daughters of women who took the drug diethylstilbestrol (DES) during pregnancy.
- Cigarette smoke, being a smoker or being around smoke.
- Women in a low socioeconomic bracket, whose living and working conditions are of poor quality, have a much higher incidence of CIN and cancers and are more likely to develop CIN at an earlier age than middle-class women due to the higher levels of stress in their lives.[8]

A healthy survey of 2,345 lesbian and bisexual women done by

Susan R. Johnson, M.D., M.S., Elaine M. Smith, Ph.D., and Susan M. Guenthe, Ph.D., confirmed "the speculation that the risk of CIN among lesbians is associated with their exposure to coitus."[9] Routine Pap smears are recommended for lesbians who were or are sexually active with men. Lesbian women who have never been active with men are encouraged to get a Pap smear every 1–3 years.

Preventive Measures

For women having intercourse with men, use a barrier method of contraception, either a condom or a diaphragm. This may help abnormal cells return to normal and prevent CIN. A report put out by the American Cancer Society says that the substances released by sperm such as arginine-rich histone or protamine may be transmissible oncogenic agents.

Reduce exposure to cigarette smoke and environmental pollutants and reduce use of oral contraceptives and immune-suppressive substances.

Dietary Support

A nourishing diet that supports and strengthens the immune system and overall health helps prevent CIN. Reduce or eliminate intake of nonorganic animal products, alcohol, caffeine, sugars, fats, fried foods, processed foods, and drugs. The key to healing is to cleanse, nourish, and support all the body's systems. This will help restore cellular integrity to the newly forming columnar epithelium tissue.

Supplements

Beta-carotene—50,000 IU, twice daily with meals

Vitamin C—2000–3000 mg two to three times per day, decrease if stools become loose

Vitamin E—400 IU per day with meals

Folic acid—2 mg per day for three months

Selenium—200 mg per day

Zinc—30 mg per day

Organic flax-seed oil—2–3 teaspoons, twice daily, mixed with grains, vegetables, or soup.

Rest

Rest, meditation, massage, acupuncture, and journal writing are some ways to reduce stress and strengthen the body. Creating time and quiet space to focus on healing is not easy for many women, given their difficult living and working situations. When possible, give yourself some space to visualize healthy vaginal cells forming.

Sitz Baths

Do a sitz bath, two to four nights per week.

Herbal Support Formula

The following herbal formula contains herbs that support the hormonal system and the liver and assist the body's ability to eliminate metabolic wastes.

> Red clover—2 parts
> Violet leaves—1 part
> Calendula—2 parts
> Dandelion root—1 part
> Cleavers—2 parts
> Licorice root—2 parts
> Thuja—1 part

Dose and Use: Place 25–50 drops of tincture in steaming hot water, let sit for five minutes, and drink 2–3 times per day for three months. Drink 1–3 cups of red clover and calendula tea daily for several weeks or months.

Immune Enhancing Herbs

These herbs are safe to take over several months for improving the health of the immune system in conjunction with the above formula.

> Codonopsis root—1 part
> Astragalus root—1 part

Schizandra berries—1 part

Ligustrum berries—1 part

(The above Chinese herbs are available at Chinese herb stores. Refer to mail-order section at the back of the book for Chinese herb sources.)

Dose and Use: Place 3–5 roots of astragalus and codonopsis and 2 tablespoons each of the berries into 1–2 quarts of water and let sit overnight, then simmer the herbs for one to two hours and drink the tea throughout the day for several months. Or take 25–50 drops of tincture, three times per day for several months.

Herbal Tea

The following herbal tea helps soothe and heal vaginal tissue and calms the nervous system. Drink 1–3 cups a day, several weeks before and after having a Pap smear or laser surgery. They help to promote cell healing and reduce scarring and inflammation. Take echinacea and goldenseal tincture a week before and after any invasive procedure along with the herbal formulas listed above and below.

Calendula—2 parts

Hawthorn berries—2 parts

Linden—1 part

Nettle—1 part

Plantain—1 part

Red clover—2 parts

Oatstraw—1 part

Violet leaf—2 parts

Dose and Use: Soak the herbs overnight in cool water and slowly warm, but do not boil, before drinking. Drink 1–3 cups per day.

Fresh Herbal Vaginal Pack

This procedure is one that herbalist David Winston has found to be useful for many women with class II Pap smears, since the herbs make better contact with the cervix than a vaginal suppository does. Take a handful of fresh chickweed, fresh calendula flowers, and fresh plantain leaves. Macerate them in a blender with ¼ teaspoon of goldenseal powder. Place the macerated herbs into a diaphragm and insert into the vagina. Leave in overnight. You may have a little leakage, but not much. Sleep on a towel. Carefully take out in the morning. If you feel there are herbs inside your vagina, gently douche with warm water. David recommends that women insert this herbal pack one night on, one night off, for several weeks if needed. Stay in good contact with your health care provider, who can monitor cell changes.

Note: This method is not a form of birth control. Discontinue use of diaphragm if your bladder becomes irritated, though for most women the spermicide jelly is the irritant and it is not being used during this procedure.

Herbal/Glycerine Suppository

The following recipe was created by herbalist and author Michael Moore, who uses these suppositories with women who have condyloma and are in the early stages of CIN.

You will need to purchase white disposable plastic vaginal molds, 3-ml size, from a pharmaceutical supplier. A pharmacist or health care provider can order the molds for you from: Apothecary Products, 11531 Rupp Drive, Burnsville, Minnesota 55337 (612) 890-1940.

To make approximately one hundred suppositories
(they will last for a few years if stored in a cool, dark place):

25 grams of pharmaceutical-grade gelatin powder (available
through a pharmacy either in bulk or powdered in
capsules)

175 ml of glycerine

3 ounces of high quality echinacea-root tincture

2 ounces of high quality calendula-flower tincture

Place the 5 ounces of tinctures into a double boiler and boil
down until 2½ ounces are left. Add in glycerine and warm
until mixture is almost steaming. Pour in gelatin powder
while continuously stirring with a whisk. Keep stirring until
the gelatin is completely dissolved—no more particles are
left in solution, and all the undissolved particles on the side
of your pan have been scraped into the solution. You will
have a brown syrup. Add 5 ml (1 tablespoon) of pure essential oil of Thuja occidentalis. Use a turkey baster to deliver
the liquid into the plastic molds. Once the liquid is solidi-
fied, the molds can be cut apart and taken off. Wrap in
waxed paper and store in a glass jar with a tight-fitting lid in
a cool, dry, and dark place.

Naturopathic Treatment

The naturopathic doctors have developed a treatment called the
escharotic treatment, which they use for cervical dysplasias and car-
cinoma *in situ*. It is a fairly involved treatment where special
enzymes and herbs are applied onto the cervix and left on for varying lengths of time and then a vaginal suppository created by the
Eclectic doctors at the turn of the century, called the vaginal depletion pack, is inserted into the vagina and left in for twenty-four
hours. The treatment is repeated several times and the protocol followed depends on the degree of dysplasia. Systemic treatment of
the immune system with various therapeutic doses of supplements

and herbs is prescribed along with suggestions for dietary and lifestyle changes and homeopathic constitutional treatment. To find a naturopathic doctor in your area who could do this treatment, contact the American Association of Naturopathic Physicians in Washington State by calling (206) 323–7610.

CONDYLOMA

Condyloma warts and the invisible (to the eye) flat lesions on the cervix are caused by the human papilloma virus (HPV). An HPV infection can be sexually transmitted, and both partners must be treated. HPV is currently being studied because of research showing possible connections to cervical cancer.

This virus may show up as abnormal cells on a Pap smear. A colposcope (a magnifying microscope) can also be used to see tiny lesions after the cervix has been bathed in acetic acid. An acid treatment and cryotherapy (freezing the warts) are common treatments for removing the warts. This often causes scarring, making the tissue sore and vulnerable.

Various forms of stress, including stress in a sexual relationship, issues of sexuality, sexual abuse, a new sexual partner, or ending a relationship, may aggravate the condition. Bringing sexual concerns into the light, talking, writing, drawing, dancing, keeping a dream journal, and doing some form of emotional release work can all be helpful therapies. I think there are stories to be told by these warts, which are usually invisible and appear in "dark, hidden, secret" places in the body.

It is important to work with an experienced and sensitive health care provider who can monitor the warts and their changes. Simple whole foods, rest, and hormonal balancing herbs, which nourish the nervous system, and immune enhancing herbs are supportive measures to incorporate into your life whether you choose to do an allopathic or natural treatment. A homeopathic constitutional may be valuable in assisting the body's healing process in conjunction with the following suggestions. Healing can occur more quickly if you avoid having fingers or a penis in your vagina.

Note: If you are pregnant seek out appropriate help with designing a treatment plan.

❀

Hormonal Balancing Formula

The following herbs help balance the hormonal system, strengthen the nervous system, and ease feelings of tension and anxiety.

St. Johnswort flowers—2 parts

Lemon balm—2 parts

Raspberry leaves—1 part

Vitex berries—2 parts

Blue vervain—1 part

Oatstraw—1 part

Dose and Use: To make a tea, steep 6 tablespoons of the herbs, covered, in a quart of hot, steaming water for ten to twenty minutes. Drink 2–4 cups per day, or take 25–50 drops of tincture, one to three times per day, for six to eight weeks.

❀

Immune Enhancing Formula

Echinacea root—2 parts

Spilanthes—1 part

Cleavers—2 parts

Usnea—1 part

Thuja—1 part

Calendula—2 parts

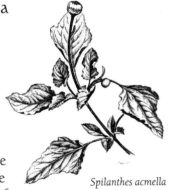

Spilanthes acmella

Dose and Use: Most effective when taken as a tincture. Place 25–50 drops into a small glass of water. Drink three times per day, five to six days a week for one month, or up to three months if needed.

SUPPLEMENTS

Vitamin C—1000–2000 mg, two to three times per day

Vitamin E—400 IU per day with meals

Beta-carotene—100,000 IU, twice per day with meals

A good quality B-complex vitamin (follow directions on bottle)

Organic flax-seed oil—2–3 teaspoons, twice daily mixed with grains, vegetables, or soup.

Oil for Topical Application

For genital warts you can see with your own eyes, herbalist Amanda McQuade Crawford recommends adding 25 drops of the pure essential oil of Thuja occidentalis to a 1-ounce bottle of herb oil made with equal parts of the following oils: calendula, St. Johns-wort, and comfrey root and leaf. Put a few drops of the oil onto a cotton swab or Q-Tip and place directly onto the wart, twice a day, four to five days a week, to help break it down. Use a speculum and have a friend with clean hands assist you.

OTHER NATURAL AIDS FOR CONDYLOMA

Consult with a naturopathic doctor, who may recommend doing a vaginal depletion pack or the escharotic treatment described under CIN.

Use the herbal/glycerine suppositories discussed under CIN.

If you have a cone biopsy or choose cryotherapy to remove the warts, follow suggestions under CIN for promoting cell healing.

CHLAMYDIA

Chlamydia trachomatis is a bacteria which was thought, before the 1970s, to be a virus. It is the most common sexually transmitted disease in developed countries. The most common sites of infection are the cervix in women and the urethra in men. Cervicitis or ure-thritis often appears seven to twenty-eight days after contact with the bacteria, but many people remain asymptomatic for years.

Untreated chlamydia can cause serious health problems for women with genital infections. Twenty percent of infections devel-op into pelvic inflammatory disease. Complications during pregnancy can also occur, including premature birth and infection of the infant.

If you have a male sex partner who has nongonococcal urethritis (NGU), you can become infected with the bacterium ureaplasma urealyticum (also called T-myocoplasma), which can be transmitted with chlamydia or separately. Ureaplasma has also been found in the genital tracts of healthy people who show no signs of infection. It is essential that sexual partners communicate honestly with each other about their past and present health so as to avoid infecting their partner with chlamydia or another sexually transmitted disease (STD).

POSSIBLE SYMPTOMS (MANY WOMEN HAVE NO SYMPTOMS)

- Painful or frequent urination
- Cervicitis (inflamed cervix)
- Cervical discharge—may be thick, yellow or greenish, although on occasion can be thin and clear
- Lower-abdominal pain
- Inflamed and sore labia
- Pain with intercourse

The new swabs for the chlamydia antibody are very effective for diagnosing. Contact your family planning center or public health department for updated research on diagnosis, new drugs, and any possible side effects.

The standard treatment today for chlamydia is doxycycline. Pregnant women must avoid doxycycline. If an infection does recur, sometimes another kind of antibiotic needs to be used. Allopathic medicine recommends regular sexual partners both be treated. If antibiotics fail there is the possibility that your infection could be another kind of bacteria or pelvic inflammatory disease (PID).

DIETARY SUPPORT

As with any infection, support the body with a simple, whole-foods diet. Reduce intake of sugar, fats, alcohol, nicotine, and processed foods. A balanced diet with grains, beans, lots of green leafy vegetables, seaweeds, root vegetables, and lots of garlic strengthens the immune system.

SUPPLEMENTS

Vitamin C—1000–3000 mg two to three times per day, up to bowel tolerance

Vitamin E—400 IU daily with meals

Beta-carotene—50,000–75,000 IU, twice daily with meals

Zinc—30 mg per day

A good quality B-complex vitamin (follow directions on bottle)

Organic flax-seed oil—2–3 teaspoons, twice daily mixed into grains, vegetables, or soup.

HERBAL SUPPORT

Seek good support from an experienced naturopathic, homeopathic, or open-minded allopathic doctor. If your infection does not respond quickly to holistic treatments you will want to discuss antibiotics with your doctor. Homeopathic constitutional treatment and herbs can be supportive even if you choose to use antibiotics.

Herbal Tincture

Goldenseal root—3 parts

Usnea—2 parts

Echinacea root—1 part

Myrrh—1 part

Dose and Use: Take 25–50 drops, three to four times per day for two to three weeks. Continue to monitor your infection with a doctor. Some naturopathic doctors use the vaginal depletion pack (described above under CIN).

Other possible herbs to take orally along with the above herbs include the following uterine tonics and hormone-balancing herbs.

Blue cohosh root—2 parts
False unicorn root—1 part
Sarsaparilla root—1 part
Vitex berries—1 part

Dose and Use: As a tincture, take 25–50 drops, three times a day. These herbs can be taken even if you are doing a course of antibiotics and continue them for another two weeks after completion of antibiotics. Many herbalists suggest taking herbs at a different time during the day than antibiotics.

Herb Wash for Sore and Inflamed Labia

Mix equal parts of calendula flowers, plantain leaves, yarrow flowers, chickweed, and comfrey leaves. Pour 1 cup of hot, steaming water over 2 tablespoons of dried herbs or a good handful of fresh herbs. Steep, covered, for thirty minutes. Strain and gently squirt tea onto labia as often as feels good.

As with any infection, good emotional support and rest are essential for healing.

HEALING FROM ABUSE

Growing up in a patriarchal system is often hurtful to women. Most women have experienced some form of direct sexual, verbal, or physical abuse. Women who have not been directly attacked are still affected by the antifemale messages portrayed in the media, in the clothing industry, in books, and in lyrics to songs. Each of us is affected in different ways, and each woman's healing journey is personal and unique. There is no one way to heal the deep fear, hurt, grief, shame, sadness, anger, rage, despair, and disbelief that many women feel. The healing process is an ongoing one that changes as the wounds heal and as we no longer view ourselves as victims.

Each time a woman stands up and refuses to be victimized, she gives courage for another woman to do the same.

I have listened to many women's stories over the years, including when I volunteered for a battered women's hotline for three years. The following herbal formulas are inspired by my own healing journey, by many other women's stories, and by the thoughtfulness of two herbalists, Hart Brent and Matty Becker. Homeopathic constitutional treatment may be helpful along with other modalities such as body work, dream therapy, dance or movement therapy, journal writing, and counseling. For many a woman, the most important piece of her healing is to make a relationship with her physical body and relearn how to love and nurture herself.

Strengthening Herbs

This formula supports anyone who has abuse memories resurfacing and feels physically and emotionally drained or stunned, or for a woman who has recently been raped or abused. It also helps people who feel overwhelmed and hopeless by the abusive situations occurring in the world.

The herbs help to clear the mental fog or numbness that usually accompanies any traumatic experience. Specifically, St. Johnswort, lavender, and rosemary support the nervous system and ease heart pain and feelings of depression. Calamus root helps deeply buried feelings rise to consciousness and be spoken of and circulates energy in the brain so one can see a situation more clearly. (The Sanskrit word for calamus is *vac*. Vac is also a Hindu goddess whose name means speech or word.) Red ginseng is specific for healing shock and fright and for restoring loss of energy and vitality. Various flower essences, specific for each person, can be taken along with any of the following herbs to calm and ease feelings of shock, fear, anxiety, and nervousness.

St. Johnswort flowers—2 parts

Lavender flowers—1 part

Rosemary—1 part

Calamus root—½ part

Red ginseng root—½ part

Dose and Use: To make a tea, simmer the roots thirty to forty minutes, add the flowers and leaves, and steep, covered, for one to four hours. Drink a cup of tea two to four times a day. Can also take in tincture form, which is easier for some women, since calamus root has an acrid taste. (If you cannot tolerate the taste of calamus root replace it with sacred basil.) Take 15–25 drops of tincture, one to three times per day.

Sleeping Herbs

Many women have difficulty sleeping when old memories are surfacing or when they are processing a disturbing or terrifying experience. The following herbs can be taken before bed and if you awake during the night. They nourish the nervous system, relax the body, and calm the mind.

Skullcap—1 part

Hops—1 part

Motherwort—1 part

Chamomile—1 part

Lemon balm—2 parts

Valerian root (include with above herbs for severe
    insomnia)—1 part

Dose and Use: To make tea, boil 1 cup of water and let 2–3 teaspoons of herbs steep, covered, five to ten minutes. If using valerian root, simmer for twenty minutes before adding the leaves and flowers. It has a strong flavor, which some people dislike. I think these herbs are easier to take in tincture form because of their bitter taste. Take 25–50 drops as needed.

Releasing Anger Herbs

The following herbs support the liver when someone is feeling angry or doing specific therapy work focused on discharging anger. These herbs nourish the liver as anger is surfacing and being released. Be sure to keep the energy moving by staying physically active and/or by receiving body work.

> Bupleurum root—2 parts
> Dandelion root—2 parts
> Dong Quai root—1 part
> Blessed thistle—1 part
> Licorice root—½ part

Dose and Use: Simmer 6–10 tablespoons of the roots for thirty to forty minutes in one quart of water, covered. Add in the blessed thistle and steep for ten minutes. Take 1 cup when needed, at least once or twice a day, over several weeks or months. If using a tincture, take 15–25 drops, one or two times per day, four to five days a week for several weeks or months.

Grounding Herbs

Lots of women find it difficult to live fully in their physical bodies. Many women learned to survive abuse and other emotionally devastating experiences by mentally leaving their bodies. The following formula contains many roots. Roots help reconnect us with Earth and with our bodies. These particular roots support and ground a person as she processes or digests tough experiences. They nourish the heart, tone the lungs, and rebuild vitality.

> Hawthorn berries—1 part
> Licorice root—½ part

Marshmallow root—1 part
Schizandra berries—2 parts
Astragalus root—2 parts
Angelica root—1 part

Dose and Use: To make tea, place 6–12 tablespoons of herbs in 1–2 quarts of water, simmer thirty to forty minutes, and steep, covered, thirty minutes to four hours. Drink 1–2 cups per day. As a tincture take 25–35 drops one to two times per day.

❀

Broken Heart Herbs

Many women experience deep sadness and grief at some point in their healing journey. The following herbs are soothing and calming to the body and spirit and have an affinity with the heart. Feeling and releasing grief is part of the healing process. As grief is released, a woman is better able to breathe life energy into her body.

Heartsease pansy

Hawthorn flowers and berries—
   2 parts
Motherwort—1 part
Lemon balm—2 parts
Heartsease pansy—1 part

Dose and Use: To make a tea, pour 1 cup of hot, steaming water over 2–4 teaspoons of herbs. Steep, covered, for ten to twenty minutes. Drink 2–4 cups per day. As a tincture, take 5–10 drops whenever needed.

Hawthorn flower essence is one of my favorite essences for helping heal a broken heart. Take as many times a day as needed.

Thyme Bath

Thyme is an herb I keep close to me when I need courage. It is a nice healing herb to add to a warm bath as often as you want when you are grieving and feeling deep sadness stirring inside.

Take 1–2 cups of dried thyme, 2–3 cups if fresh, and pour 3–4 quarts of boiling water over the leaves and steep, covered, for fifteen to thirty minutes. Strain and add to your warm bathwater and soak for twenty minutes. Do every night for two weeks when you are in active stages of grieving.

Gladdening the Heart Herbs

Various herbs and flower essences help return the spark of life into our eyes and feelings of joy after we have released some of the initial pain and anguish. Spending time with the natural world, learning to move harmoniously with the seasons and the moon, and making relationships with herbs, flowers, and trees are some ways that help us feel the interconnectedness of all life. As we heal, we reenter our bodies and the web of life and are once again able to feel alive. The following herbs are easy to grow in your garden and are ones that feel joyful and nourishing to me. Add in other herbs that feel joyful to you.

Comfrey flowers

Heartsease pansy flowers

Calendula flowers

Sacred basil leaves and flowers

Lady's mantle flowers and leaves
Borage flowers and leaves
Lemon balm flowers and leaves
Bee balm flowers

Dose and Use: To make a summer tea, place whatever pro-portions of these fresh herbs or others you have into cool water and let them infuse in the sunlight or moonlight or slowly heat to near boiling and steep, covered, ten minutes. Drink 2–4 cups a day. You can dry any of these herbs or place them fresh in a jar and make a tincture for winter use.

Much healing happens when we take time each day to be present with the beauty around us and to touch with love and tenderness what once was wounded by hatred, fear, and anger. Love, kindness, and compassion are strong medicine.

9

We Are More Than Uteruses and Breasts

Women cannot have control over our own lives until we have control over our own bodies; thus understanding and gaining control over our bodies and our health is essential to taking control of our lives.[1]

—WOMEN'S HEALTH READINGS ON SOCIAL, ECONOMICAL, AND POLITICAL ISSUES

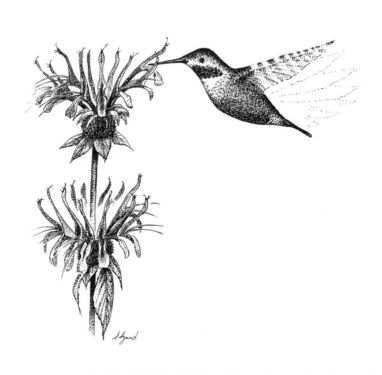

*S*ome health care providers view women's health as having only to do with the health of our reproductive organs and breasts. Even though these areas in our bodies sometimes require extra attention, their health is dependent on the health of the whole body. This chapter includes herbal and nutritional support for various health conditions, some of which are related to our abdominal area. Also included is a section on health for lesbian and bisexual women.

ENDOMETRIOSIS

Endometriosis is a condition whose cause is unknown to the modern medical world. The endometrial tissue, which normally lines the uterus, grows outside the uterine cavity. Usually the tissue starts to grow on the ovaries or fallopian tubes. The abnormal tissue and growths bleed during menstruation as they are affected by the hormonal changes of the menstrual cycle. This blood is unable to leave the body and can cause mild to severe inflammation, bleeding, cysts, and scar tissue.

Some of the symptoms that can be associated with endometriosis are: severe pelvic pain during menstruation, unusually heavy menstrual bleeding, irregular periods, infertility, a higher than average rate of miscarriage, feelings of exhaustion, and pain during ovulation or with sexual intercourse. There is an increased risk of an ectopic pregnancy for women with endometriosis.

A pelvic exam can reveal if the ovaries are swollen and the uterus is tender. Most physicians recommend a laparoscopy to make a definite diagnosis. This surgical procedure does involve some risks. Be sure to go over these with your doctor. If you go ahead with the procedure, take homeopathic arnica pills, 30c (available through health food stores and mail order), two to three times the day before, the day of, and the day after the procedure to lessen feelings of pain and bruising. Then take homeopathic *Bellis peren-*

nis, 30c, two to three times a day for a few days to help the tissue heal.

TREATMENTS

Options offered by Western medicine for treating endometriosis include: creating an anovulatory cycle, a cycle in which a woman does not release an egg; contraceptives; surgical removal of the displaced excess endometrial tissue (in severe cases a hysterectomy

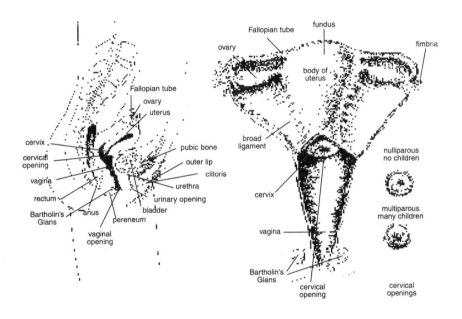

may be recommended); or the drug Danazol, which suppresses the pituitary-ovarian axis and in turn alters the hormonal feedback loop that regulates the menstrual cycle.

Holistic therapies such as herbs, homeopathy, and acupuncture have been shown to be effective in reducing pain and excessive bleeding and increasing overall health for some women. The vital force within each of us becomes stronger when supportive therapies are used. Rebuilding the body's overall strength takes time, however. Herbs and other modalities do not offer a quick fix. Patience, trust, love, and a commitment to your healing process are needed. If you observe little improvement in your health over two to four months, reevaluate your health plan with an experienced practitioner.

Many factors are involved with choosing a treatment. Diet, acupuncture, chiropractic and/or cranial-sacral adjustments (very subtle adjustments of the cranial bones), homeopathy, counseling, deep emotional cleansing work, and dream therapy are possible avenues to explore, but they can be expensive. Listen to the deeper messages your body gives you and find people you feel safe with to assist you. Some of the emotional areas to consider may include looking at your relationship with your womb. How do you feel about your body? What is/was your relationship with your mother, your grandmother, or past and/or present lovers? Have you ever been pregnant, miscarried, or had an abortion? Do you have children, do you want children, or do you have lingering feelings about not having children? When possible, create quiet moments to focus on yourself and your healing journey.

DIETARY SUPPORT

Whether you choose surgery, drugs, or herbs, a nourishing diet with herbs that tone the uterus, liver, and the hormonal and nervous systems is important for supporting the body's ability to heal. If you decide to have surgery, diet and herbs can still help support the healing process. If you are taking Danazol or another drug, be sure to also take herbs that support the liver and immune system. The dietary suggestions and supplements listed below are helpful whether you choose to have surgery or not.

- Decrease intake of fatty foods, including dairy products, as much as possible. The estrogen present in dairy products encourages the growth of endometrial tissue.

- Reduce or eliminate meat or chicken that has been injected with hormones and avoid eggs from commercial houses whenever possible.

- Endometriosis is a condition in which the energy in the pelvic area is slow moving. Avoid eating and drinking cold foods and beverages. Eat warm foods before eating a salad or fruit.

SUPPLEMENTS

Vitamin E—200 IU, twice daily with meals, helps keep scar tissue soft and flexible (Take 100 IU daily if you have high blood pressure.)

Vitamin C—1000–2000 mg, take two to three times a day with meals

Beta-carotene—50,000 IU, twice daily

A good quality B-complex vitamin with extra folic acid and B6

Organic flax-seed oil—2–3 teaspoons, twice daily, mixed into vegetables or grain. Flax-seed oil contains linoleic acid (Omega-6 family) and linolenic acids (Omega-3 family), which regulate prostaglandin production. Prostaglandins are hormonelike chemicals that have many functions, including regulating pain and inflammation

Drink a cup of yellow dock root and nettle tea, two to three times daily or take a tincture of these two herbs, 25–50 drops, two to three times daily, for increasing iron, or use a commercially prepared product called Floradix, which is available through most health food stores.

Liver Support Herbs

Include foods such as beets and carrots in your diet and drink a few cups of water with freshly squeezed lemon daily for improving liver health. Use the following herbs as a daily tonic:

Dandelion root—2 parts
Blessed thistle—2 parts
Wild yam root—1 part
Milk thistle seed—1 part
Chicory root—1 part

Dose and Use: Take as a tincture, 25–50 drops, in a small glass of water, two to three times per day before meals, for two to three months. After three months reevaluate your health plan and continue with liver herbs as needed.

Hormonal Support Herbs

There is no one magic herb formula that heals endometriosis. Each woman's body and circumstances are unique and must be considered when designing an herbal formula. The following herbs help regulate hormonal balance, improve the health of uterine tissue, and bring blood to the pelvic area.

White ash bark—2 parts

Saw palmetto berries—1 part

Vitex berries—4 parts

False unicorn root—1 part

Dose and Use: Take as a tincture, 1 tsp., in a small glass of water, three times a day, for two to three months and longer if needed. You can take these herbs with the above liver herbs.

Easing Pain Herbs

For acute pain use the following herbal remedy:

Valerian root—1 part

Crampbark—1 part

Black cohosh root—1 part

Wild yam root—1 part

Dose and Use: Take 30–60 drops of tincture, as needed, for relieving acute pain.

Other Supportive Therapies for Easing Pain

Yoga, massage, polarity therapy, acupuncture, meditation, and visualization also help relieve pain. Sitz baths, four to five per week, help improve circulation to the pelvic area, as does doing daily Kegel exercises (tightening and releasing the pubococcygeus muscle, the muscle that stops urination, consistently starting with 10–20, two to three times a day and working up to a total of 200 a day).

Nervous System Tonic

Living with physical pain on a daily basis wears down the nervous system. The following herbs, taken as tea or tincture, help relax the body, nourish the nervous system, and contain minerals for promoting overall health.

Oatstraw—2 parts

Skullcap—1 part

Lavender—1 part

Linden flowers and leaves—2 parts

Lemon balm—2 parts

Horsetail—1 part

Nettle—1 part

Dose and Use: To make tea, place 4–6 tablespoons of herbs in a pint or quart glass jar and pour 2–4 cups of hot water into the jar, cover, and let steep for five to ten minutes or longer. You can also let 4–6 tablespoons of herbs sit in a pot with 2–4 cups of cool water overnight and the next morning slowly warm up the tea, take off the heat, and steep for another five to ten minutes. Strain the herbs. Drink 1–3 cups daily or take 25–50 drops of tincture, two to three times daily.

Herbs for Heavy Bleeding

If you are prone to heavy bleeding when you menstruate, the following remedy will help ease the flow.

Fresh shepherd's purse—3 parts
Bethroot—1 part
Lady's mantle flowers and leaves—1 part
Yarrow flowers—2 parts

Dose and Use: Take the tincture two to three days before you bleed, 20–25 drops, three to four times per day. You can take 40–50 drops of tincture as needed if bleeding is heavy. If your bleeding is severe and continuous seek appropriate help. Be sure to take herbs and eat food high in iron on a daily basis, because iron is lost through blood.

Belly Oil

Create a special oil to rub onto your belly after baths and/or before sleeping to ensure a free flow of energy throughout your womb area. Add 3–4 drops of each of the following essential oils, sweet marjoram, ginger, and sassafras, into an ounce of vegetable oil such as almond, apricot kernel, olive, or grape-seed oil.

Castor-oil Packs

Castor-oil packs improve circulation, ease pain, and break up congestion. Use three to five times a week before bed. Do not use a castor-oil pack when menstruating. (See directions in chapter 2.)

Note: It is best not to use tampons or an IUD and avoid X-rays if you have endometriosis.

The Endometriosis Association is a national self-help organization formed in 1980 whose goals include: supporting and helping women with endometriosis, educating the public and medical community, and doing research. They offer a newsletter, crisis telephone services, support meetings around the United States, and literature. For more information, write to the Endometriosis Association, 8585 North 76th Place, Milwaukee, WI 53223, or call (800) 992-3636, in the United States, and (800) 426-2363, in Canada.

OVARIAN CYSTS

Ovarian cysts are a common occurrence in women and often present no symptoms. They appear when a follicle has grown large and failed to rupture and release an egg. Most of these cysts are filled with fluid and are called functional cysts and often disappear by themselves. If they become solid they are usually referred to as tumors, which can be either benign or malignant.

If a woman has unfamiliar pain in the lower abdomen, abdominal swelling, or severe fluctuations in her menstrual cycle, a routine pelvic exam or pelvic ultrasound may, but not always, reveal cysts. Sometimes a cyst can suddenly decide to surprise a woman and burst, causing excruciating pain in the area where the ovary is located.

I had five ovarian cysts burst over a period of nine months in 1993. What follows is my personal story with cysts. Other women's experiences with cysts may be quite different. I never knew I had a cyst until one morning in April when I was driving home from the car mechanic and I suddenly doubled over in pain. The pain felt like the worst menstrual cramps I had ever experienced.

I crawled up the stairs to my bedroom and lay on my bed crying in pain. I kept saying that my ovary felt like it was bursting. I wanted to get out of my physical body. My partner Abby helped me stay focused on breathing and massaged my feet. After about forty-five minutes the pain began to subside and I fell asleep. Two doctor friends returned my phone calls in the afternoon and verified that a cyst had burst. Both my ovaries felt extremely tender, like someone had punched me. My doctor suggested I take the homeopathic remedy, *Bellis perennis*, (English daisy), which is specific for bruised feelings in the ovaries. It worked. The bruised feelings subsided within twenty minutes after taking one 30c dose. Castor-oil packs also helped ease the pain.

My journey with cysts continued. They all have burst two to four days after I finished menstruating. Homeopathic colocynthis, 30c, helped ease the initial doubling-over pain each time. I then took *Bellis perennis*, 30c, two to three times a day over the next few days and did a castor-oil pack for a few nights, both of which felt soothing and took away the pain.

My inner journey with understanding cysts continues to change and evolve with time. Over these months I have begun to view my ovaries, uterus, and breasts as organs for receiving deep, intuitive messages from the depths of my psyche—my ovaries are eyes to help me see in the dark. The sudden explosive quality of a cyst bursting gets my attention fast. I continue to ask for help in understanding what my cysts are trying to communicate to me during meditation and through dreams.

TREATMENT

Medical professionals often suggest watching what a cyst does for a few cycles before recommending treatment, which may include oral contraceptives. Once it is determined that a painful cyst is nonmalignant and not causing any serious health complications, herbs, homeopathy, and dietary support can be effective in reducing or dissolving the cyst, decreasing the size of the ovary, and bringing the hormonal system into balance. Addressing stressful areas can also be helpful in preventing functional cysts from recurring. If they do recur, seek appropriate medical care.

DIETARY SUPPORT

Follow a simple whole foods diet that includes brown rice and lots of dark leafy green vegetables such as kale and collards; root vegetables such as carrots, beets, burdock, and onions; seaweeds; and seasonal fruits. Keep your intake of carbohydrates to a minimum. Eat as much kelp as possible, cooked in soups or in your grains, vegetables, salads, and dressings, or take in tablet form if you can't stand to eat it. Reduce or eliminate coffee, alcohol, chocolate, sugar, and white flour.

SUPPLEMENTS

Beta-carotene—50,000 IU, twice daily

Vitamin C—1000–2000 mg, two to three times a day with meals

Vitamin E—400 IU, daily with meals

Zinc—25–30 mg daily

Essential fatty acids–Mix 2–3 teaspoons of flax-seed oil with steamed vegetables, soups, or cooked grain, twice daily

Herbs for Relieving Acute Ovarian Pain

Passion flower—1 part

Valerian root—2 parts

Crampbark—1 part

Skullcap—1 part

Yellow birch twigs—2 parts

False unicorn root—2 parts

Dose and Use: Take as a tincture, 25–50 drops, every hour, or as needed to ease pain.

Herbs for Reducing and Dissolving Cysts

Chickweed—1 part

Vitex berries—3 parts

Redroot—2 parts

Violet leaves—1 part

Cleavers—2 parts

Blue cohosh root—1 part
White ash bark—3 parts

Dose and Use: Take in tincture form, 25–50 drops, three to four times per day for two to four months. The nourishing and mineral-rich tea listed under endometriosis is a good tea to drink on a daily basis along with taking the hormonal support herbs listed under endometriosis.

Liver Support Herbs

A healthy liver plays an important role in reducing ovarian cysts and eliminating various waste products.

Dandelion root—2 parts
Blessed thistle—1 part
Yellow dock root—1 part
Milk thistle seed—1 part
Wild yam root—2 parts

Dose and Use: Take as a tincture, 20–40 drops before meals, two to three times daily for one to three months. Keep assessing the health of your liver and continue with liver support herbs and food in some routine way that works with your overall health plan.

Corsican Sea Vegetable Tea

This tea is a macrobiotic remedy for dissolving ovarian cysts and uterine fibroids. The tea is very mucilaginous. Take 5–10 grams of dried seaweed. Simmer for ten to twenty minutes in 2 cups of water and drink daily. You may have to give yourself a pep talk before drinking this slimy tea.

POST-SURGICAL SUPPORT

If the cyst is removed surgically, follow guidelines listed under hysterectomy for herbal support.

ADDITIONAL SUPPORT FOR PREVENTING CYSTS

- Castor-oil packs over the sore ovary, two to five nights a week.
- Alternating hot and cold sitz baths daily or as often as you can.
- Yoga, which supports the endocrine glands and increases circulation to the pelvis.
- Cranial-sacral manipulation, which improves energy flow to the pelvic area and realigns the whole body.
- Meditation and prayer.
- Deep breathing.
- Flower essences.
- Creative movement.
- Drawing and journal writing.
- Learning to just be.

UTERINE FIBROIDS

Fibroids are solid, noncancerous growths that usually appear on the inside of the uterus, though they can also grow on the outside of the uterus. Fibroids are called benign tumors by Western medical doctors. Over 90 percent of these so-called tumors are nonmalignant.[2]

Allopathic medicine does not know the cause of fibroids. They can be tiny or as large as grapefruits. The smaller ones are usually symptomless. Larger ones can cause heavy menstrual bleeding or bleeding between periods, abdominal and lower-back pain, and urinary problems. Large fibroids can also create problems when trying to conceive or when carrying a baby to full term. Their growth is accelerated by estrogenic foods (meat and dairy), a weak liver, poor elimination, an increase of estrogen levels from oral contraceptives, estrogen replacement therapies, and pregnancy.

Fibroids can be found during a pelvic exam. Having them checked every three to six months by a health care provider is a way to monitor their size. There is usually no need for surgery unless the fibroids are causing health complications. A surgical procedure called a myomectomy removes the fibroid and leaves the uterus. A hysterectomy removes the uterus and sometimes the ovaries. Be sure to get a second opinion when considering surgery.

TREATMENT

Uterine fibroids can be a sign of poor circulation in the pelvic area. Some of the following suggestions can help improve circulation to the pelvis.

- Breathing deeply into your womb several times a day. Doing daily Kegel exercises and yoga, especially the pelvic rock, encourages circulation into the pelvic area.
- Several sitz baths weekly will stimulate the flow of energy to the pelvis.
- Orgasms help energy to flow.
- Castor-oil packs, placed over the fibroid three to four times per week, may help decrease the size of fibroids and improve pelvic circulation.
- Poke root oil massaged over the fibroid nightly.
- Herbalist Tiearona Klar Low Dog has seen good results using a cooked down chaparral mixture for reducing fibroids. She works in an herbal clinic in Albuquerque, New Mexico. For purchasing the chaparral mixture call the clinic at (505) 255-9215.
- Various kinds of body work such as acupuncture and shiatsu massage also increase energy flow and relieve pain.

Some women say that being in a dialogue with their fibroid has helped them listen to the story their body wants to tell. This communication happens more easily when you let yourself be in a meditative or relaxed state. If you work with your dreams, ask them for help each night before bed. Daily or weekly journal writing and drawing can be helpful avenues for letting your inner self come out. Focus on your own healing in the ways you feel drawn to. I believe part of every woman's healing journey is learning to not blame herself for whatever health condition she may be facing.

DIETARY SUPPORT

A simple whole foods diet, high in dark leafy green vegetables, sea vegetables (especially kelp and corsican seaweed tea), and various whole grains strengthens and reenergizes the body. Avoid cold foods; they aggravate poor circulation.

Fibroids are estrogen dependent. A diet low in estrogenic substances—dairy products, and nonorganic meat and chicken and eggs—helps reduce fibroids. As you can, eliminate coffee; decaffeinated coffee; chocolate; black teas; alcohol, especially beer (beer contains hops and hops contain estrogenic substances); aspirin; and nicotine.

If your digestion is slow and sluggish, or too active, follow the suggestions in chapter 5. Dietary changes, physical movement, herbs, and emotional healing can help with constipation.

SUPPLEMENTS

Vitamin C—1000–2000 mg, three times a day with meals

Vitamin E—400 IU, once a day with meals

Beta-carotene—50,000 IU, twice daily

Zinc—30 mg per day

Selenium—200 mg per day

Organic flax-seed oil—2–3 teaspoons, twice daily, mixed with grains, vegetables, or salad. Helps ease muscle cramps and tension and reduce inflamed tissues.

Herbal Support

The liver is involved with processing estrogen and keeping estrogen levels balanced. Include liver-supporting foods such as carrots and beets on a regular basis along with the following herbs.

Dandelion root—2 parts

Blessed thistle—1 part

Wild yam root—1 part
Milk thistle seed—1 part
Burdock root—2 parts

Dose and Use: Take 25–50 drops of tincture, two to three times a day before meals, for several weeks.

Herbs for Balancing Hormones

The following formula can be taken two to four times per day, five times per week, over several months, to help reduce fibroids, relieve inflammation, and regulate hormone levels.

Vitex berries (chasteberry)—2 parts
Saw palmetto berries—1 part
Black cohosh root—1 part
Blue cohosh root—2 parts
Partridgeberry—1 part
White ash bark—2 parts
Cleavers—1 part

Dose and Use: Take as a tincture, 25–50 drops, two to four times per day with meals, four to five times a week, over several months.

Corsican Sea Vegetable Tea (Digenea simplex)

This tea is a macrobiotic remedy for dissolving uterine fibroids. It is very mucilagenous. Take 5–10 grams of dried seaweed and simmer for ten to twenty minutes in 2 cups of water and drink daily.

Large fibroids can be stubborn and for some women may not decrease until menopause. If you are experiencing pain and other health problems seek help from an experienced health practitioner. Talk about your feelings. If you decide to have surgery, take homeopathic arnica, 30c, two to three times the day before, the day of, and one to two days after surgery. Then take homeopathic *Bellis perennis*, 30c, two to three times a day for supporting the healing process. Have a friend organize people to bring nourishing food into the hospital for you. Follow the herbal support guidelines listed below under hysterectomy for postsurgical support.

A friend of mine who was diagnosed with a grapefruit-size fibroid found that her energy levels improved enormously and her emotions stablized with help from acupuncture and Chinese herbs that the acupuncturist prescribed for her. She is currently following a health plan outlined for her by a doctor who practices anthroposophic medicine and uses very specific homeopathic preparations. (Anthroposophic medicine was inspired by Rudolph Steiner, who was also instrumental in creating biodynamic farming practices. Refer to resource list for contacts.) My friend says her health continues to improve.

HYSTERECTOMY

Close to one million hysterectomies, removal of the uterus, are performed each year in the United States. Many of these hysterectomies are unnecessary. Surgeons often recommend a hysterectomy to fix an ongoing gynecological problem or to prevent uterine or ovarian cancer. If you or someone you know has been recommended to have a hysterectomy, get a second opinion if you are financially able. Ask lots of questions. Discuss the details of surgery with the surgeon beforehand, especially stressing to her or him to leave the ovaries if possible.

Hysterectomies are necessary when a condition is life threatening, such as invasive cancer of the uterus, cervix, vagina, or fallopian tubes, for severe pelvic inflammatory disease (PID), for uncontrollable bleeding, and for painful and debilitating conditions such as large fibroid tumors or extensive endometriosis.

Hysterectomies are sometimes used as a form of sterilization abuse against low-income women, women of color, and in some prisons in the United States and internationally. Women of color experience twice as many hysterectomies as white women in the United States.[3] Sterilizing any woman without her consent is an abusive violation. Investigate your local clinic or hospital to see if they know what the federal sterilization law says (it was passed in 1979) and ask them how they enforce it.

Presurgery

Take arnica homeopathic pills, 30c, two to three times a day, the day before, the day of, and two days after surgery to lessen the shock of surgery and to ease feelings of bruising and pain. If you have an emergency hysterectomy, take the pills as soon after the surgery as possible. Have a friend quietly put the pills under your tongue. Arnica will not interfere with any medication you may be on. Wait fifteen minutes before or after eating, drinking, or taking medications before taking arnica. Take homeopathic *Bellis perennis*, 30c, two to three times a day starting two or three days following surgery.

Postsurgical Support

- Eat foods high in bioflavanoids, such as blueberries, blackberries, hawthorn berries, and rose hips
- Vitamin C—1000–2000 mg, three times a day
- Vitamin E—400 IU per day with meals
- Beta-carotene—50,000 IU, twice daily
- Zinc—15 mg daily
- Organic flax-seed oil—2–3 teaspoons, twice daily, added to vegetables, grains, or soup

Herbal Support

Take echinacea root tea or tincture for two weeks following surgery. Echinacea will strengthen your immune system quickly and help prevent other infections.

Dose and Use: To make tea, simmer 6 tablespoons of root in one quart of water for thirty minutes. Drink 3–5 cups a day, or take 25–50 drops of tincture three to five times per day.

Mineral-Rich Tea

The following mineral-rich herbs nourish and strengthen the body.

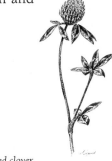

Red clover—2 parts

Calendula—2 parts

Oatstraw—1 part

Cleavers—1 part

Nettle—1 part

Raspberry leaf—1 part

Horsetail—1 part

Red clover

Dose and Use: Place 6 tablespoons of herbs in 1 quart of cool water and let steep overnight. Slowly warm the following morning. Take off the heat and steep, covered, five to ten minutes. Take this tea, 2–3 cups a day, for several weeks, along with the suggested supplements and hormonal tonic listed below for supporting the body's healing process.

Hormonal and Immune System Tonic

The following herbs strengthen the hormonal and immune systems.

Dong Quai root—2 parts

Lady's mantle—1 part

Saw palmetto berries—1 part

Siberian ginseng root—2 parts

Vitex berries—2 parts

Dandelion root—1 part

Corn silk—1 part (Delete if the urinary tract was not traumatized)

Vitex berries and Siberian ginseng influence the endocrine system and support the body through this major hormonal transition. Dong Quai and lady's mantle bring blood to the pelvic area, which helps repair damaged cells. Dong Quai also assists with the hormonal changes (hormones circulate in blood) by ensuring the blood is circulating well to the pelvic area and by facilitating the healthy functioning of the hormonal receptor sites. Saw palmetto berries help regulate hormonal balance, rebuild strength and energy, ease inflammation, and aid digestion. Dandelion is included because it helps the liver to eliminate drugs from the body. Corn silk soothes any irritation of the urinary tract (50 percent of women experience a urinary tract infection post surgically).[4]

Dose and Use: Take 25–50 drops of tincture three times a day for three to six months. Reevaluate your health needs after six months. You may want to continue with herbs for hormonal support, four to five times a week, for several more months. (Refer to section on menopause.)

If the ovaries are removed along with the uterus, add the herbs listed below to the above formula. They add extra support to the adrenal glands. The adrenal glands will continue to secrete small amounts of estrogen. If you know your ovaries will be removed before surgery occurs, begin taking the herbs listed below one to two months before surgery.

Licorice root—½ part

Sarsaparilla root—1 part

Wild yam root—1 part

Dose and Use: To make a tea, simmer the roots, covered, for thirty minutes. Drink 2–3 cups per day or take 25–35 drops of tincture three times per day.

Losing part of your body can be emotionally traumatic. Nourishing support from women friends, a partner if you are in a relationship, and close family members is essential for many women in their healing process. Flower essences, acupuncture, counseling, massage, and other healing therapies also assist in healing.

BENIGN BREAST CONDITION

Women growing up in Western cultures experience a range of feelings about their breasts. Women's bodies, especially our breasts, are used by the media and commonly highlighted on billboards and in magazines to sell tools, cigarettes, clothes, and cars. The sexually abusive display of women's breasts makes it difficult for many women to see their breasts as part of their body.

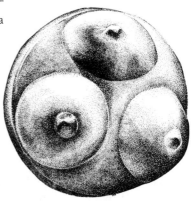

"Breast Bowl." A precolumbian bowl with a three-breasted base. "When we honor the Sacred Feminine and the Goddess, we are fed. Source of life-sustaining food and warmth, identified with the comforting sound of the heartbeat, the breast is reassurance to the abundance of the Earth Mother and of life itself." North American, 6th century C.E. (Drawn from a photograph from *The Heart of the Goddess: Art, Myth and Meditations of the World's Sacred Feminine* by Hallie Iglehart Austen, Berkeley: Wingbow Press, 1990, p. 24–25.)

Fear of getting breast cancer also gets in the way of women enjoying their breasts and doing a self-breast massage at least once a month. Many women never touch their breasts and are terrified of finding a lump that could be cancerous. It is scary that medical statistics state that now one in eight women will get breast cancer. This risk is higher if you have a mother or sister with breast cancer. Having lumpy breasts, a breast infection, nipple discharge, or finding a lump causes panic in many women. Getting acquainted with our breasts through regular breast massage, noting their changes through several menstrual cycles, and being in contact with a good health care provider who can monitor our breast changes and answer our questions is helpful in relieving anxiety. *Dr. Susan Love's Breast Book* is a useful resource book for helping to demystify breasts and for giving information on Western medical treatments for various breast conditions.

Hormonal fluctuations during ovulation, before menstruation, and during menopause can cause the breast cells to retain fluid. Many women experience lumpiness and some discomfort during different phases of their menstrual cycle. These kinds of lumps are called breast cysts and are fluid-filled sacs. They often feel sore and usually decrease in size or disappear a few days after the menstrual flow begins. Some women have localized lumps, which are solid masses of noncancerous tissue. Often a breast biopsy is recommended to distinguish these from a breast cancer. If you decide to have a biopsy, take homeopathic *Bellis perennis*, 30c, two to three times a day for a few days following the biopsy to ease bruising and help the disturbed tissue heal.

Keep a journal each month, noting when lumps appear and disappear, what kinds of foods you are eating, and specific stresses you may be experiencing. After tracking this information for a few months, you may begin to see patterns that will help you make appropriate dietary and lifestyle changes.

An annual breast exam by an experienced practitioner is recommended health maintenance for all women. If you find a lump that persists for more than one menstrual cycle, or other worrisome changes, such as nipple discharge, an evaluation by a practitioner is advisable to rule out breast cancer. It is recommended that postmenopausal women consult a practitioner for any breast lumps, skin changes, or nipple discharges since the risk of breast cancer is higher for postmenopausal women.

DIETARY SUPPORT

Reducing and eliminating caffeine, chocolate, sodas, dairy products, alcohol, fatty foods, and meat seems to help some women's cysts shrink or disappear. Include lots of dark leafy green vegetables, sea vegetables, (refer to chapter 4 for more information on breast health and sea vegetables), grains, beans, and some seasonal fruits. The National Cancer Institute and the National Academy of Sciences are currently documenting the connection of breast cancer with high fat diets. Meat and dairy products make up 40 percent of a standard American diet. These organizations both recommend a low fat diet as a cancer preventive measure.

A diet high in animal proteins and fats, overrefined, over-cooked, and rich foods weakens the digestive system, the liver, and elimination channels. When circulation is poor, the exchanges that occur on a cellular level involved with eliminating normal waste products from the cells slow down. This can cause abnormal tissues to grow in the body. Tight clothing, a sedentary lifestyle, and high stress levels also interfere with healthy digestion and elimination. If you have a tendency toward constipation, dietary changes and exercise can help, along with taking bitter tasting herbs such as gentian root, blessed thistle, burdock root with a touch of licorice, and ginger root for several weeks. (Refer to chapter 5 on how to use bitter herbs.)

SUPPLEMENTS

Vitamin C—1000–2000 mg, taken two to three times a day with meals

Beta-carotene—25,000 IU, twice daily

Vitamin E—400 IU daily with meals (buy D-alpha tocopherol)

A good quality B-complex vitamin

Organic flax-seed oil—2–3 teaspoons, twice daily mixed with grains, vegetables, or soup.

HERBAL SUPPORT

Because the fluctuations of hormones come into play with the formation of cysts, strengthening the liver with liver-tonic herbs helps support good digestion and the healthy circulation of hormones. Equal parts of dandelion root, blue vervain, and milk thistle seed tincture, taken twice a day before meals, four to five times a week, for several weeks or months can be helpful for decreasing cysts and lumps and easing soreness.

Herbal Tea

The following herbal tea contains nourishing and mineral-rich herbs for supporting overall health.

Red raspberry leaf—1 part

Red clover—2 parts

Nettle—1 part

Calendula—2 parts

Mullein leaves—1 part

Oatstraw—1 part

Lemon balm—2 parts

Dose and Use: Place 6 tablespoons of herbs in a glass quart jar and cover with hot, steaming water and let steep, covered, ten to fifteen minutes. Drink warm or cool throughout the day, four to five times a week.

HERBS FOR DECREASING BREAST CYSTS

The following formula taken in conjuction with the liver herbs and tea listed above is helpful for decreasing breast cysts or fibrocystic tissue by balancing the hormonal system and improving lymphatic drainage.

Calendula flowers–2 parts

Cleavers–1 part

Dong Quai root–1 part

Astragalus root–1 part

Violet leaves–2 parts

Vitex berries–2 parts

Dose and Use: As a tincture, take 25–50 drops, three times per day, for several weeks.

Poke Root

Poke root is specific for decreasing growths. Best to take as tincture, 2–3 drops once a day. After using for one week increase to 5 drops. Then increase to 8 drops the next week and continue taking 8 drops per day for another week. Use the poke in conjuction with the herbs listed above. If you are using poke, consult an experienced herbalist or other health care provider for assistance in reevaluating your health plan after a month.

Note: Large doses of poke can be toxic. Keep poke away from children and animals.

Dietary and herbal support may reduce the cyst or fibrocystic tissue in one cycle or may take a few months. Once they have been eliminated, be sure to continue using liver-tonic herbs, three to four times a week, and follow a good diet to prevent their return. If no changes occur after a few months, seek good help for further exploration.

Breast tissue is susceptible to cell damage through X rays. Avoid X rays when pregnant and nursing and during puberty. Be sure breasts are well shielded during dental and other X rays. Take echinacea root, astragalus root, and thuja tinctures twice a day, one week before and one week after receiving any forms of X rays, including before and after having a mammogram. Check with an informed health care provider on Western medicine's recommendations for mammograms, as they are currently changing them. Eat miso soup and seaweeds regularly to further prevent damage to the body from any form of radiation.

EXTERNAL HERBS FOR BENIGN BREAST CONDITIONS

If you have breast cancer seek guidance on the use of herbs and compresses from an experienced health care provider.

Castor-oil Packs: Use three to five times a week for three weeks. Rest a week and repeat again if needed.

Clay Poultice: Clay has a drawing action. Green clay or bentonite clay are available for sale in many health food stores. Mix the powdered clay with a small amount of water. First apply a towel soaked in hot water over the cyst or lump for five minutes. This will help improve circulation to the area. Then place the clay paste, one-half-inch thick over the area on the breast where the growth is. Leave on overnight or for three to four hours. The clay dries and can be gently removed by placing a warm, moist towel over the area. Apply once a day for a month. Clay draws the fatty mucus and other substances from the growth to the surface of the skin so that it will drain.

Poke Root Oil: Warm poke root oil can be applied over the area where the growth is every night for a month.

Breast Massage Oil: I created a Woman's Breast Massage Oil for Avena Botanicals so we could offer women something special to use when they did a regular self-breast massage. Calendula oil makes a good base for any breast oil because it helps improve lymphatic circulation. We add 2–3 drops of the pure essential oil of geranium to a 1-ounce bottle of oil. Geranium eases breast tenderness and helps relax the whole body. Happy massaging.

Urinary Tract Infections (UTI)

An infection of part of the urinary system or large numbers of microbes detected in the urine is labeled a urinary tract infection (UTI). These infections, usually caused by bacteria that travel from the colon or skin to the urethra and bladder, are common among women. Sometimes the bacteria travel to the kidneys, causing a kidney infection, a situation that needs appropriate medical attention. A poor diet, stress, an increase in sexual activity, a new sexual partner, pregnancy, surgery, catheterization, chlamydia, and trichomonas are some causes of UTI's.

Women who have birthed many children are prone to infections if their urethras or bladders are prolapsed. Postmenopausal women sometimes experience infections due to hormonal changes. Women who were made to hold their urine for long lengths of time as children, not allowed to go to the bathroom at home or at school when needed, shamed by parents or other adults about urinating, or sexually abused as children or adults, often have weakened kidneys and bladders and are susceptible to infections.

Cystitis, an inflammation or infection of the lining and wall of the bladder, is the most common UTI for women. Symptoms may include a need to urinate frequently with little urine coming out, a burning sensation during urination, or pain above the pubic bone. (Some women urinate frequently—but do not have an infection—because of a high intake of coffee or tea, food allergies, irritation from soaps, douches, nervousness, and premenstrual stress.)[5] If the symptoms continue for more than twenty-four hours and include a fever, vomiting, pain in the kidney area, and blood or pus in the urine, then you may have a kidney infection and will need to consult a trusted health care provider for assistance.

PREVENTION OF UTI

- Wipe yourself from front to back after urinating or having a bowel movement.
- Empty your bladder as often as you need.
- Drink unchlorinated water that is room temperature whenever possible. Drink an eight-ounce glass of water at least two to four times a day, and more if infection is present. Water helps to flush out bacteria. Caffeinated beverages and foods, black teas, alcohol, and nicotine irritate the bladder. Reduce your intake or eliminate them as you can.
- Foods high in sugars and white flours, as well as breads, pastas, sweetened fruit juices, or fruit juices made from concentrates, feed the unwanted bacteria.
- Empty your bladder before and after sexual activity. Be aware of sexual activity that irritates the urethra and puts pressure on the bladder. For women who use a diaphragm, be sure it fits you and the rim does not press on your urethra. Birth control pills and various contraceptive foams or suppositories can irritate the urethra. A dry condom also puts pressure on the urethra, as do tampons.
- If you use sanitary pads during your menstrual flow, change

the pad often enough to prevent the spread of bacteria from your anus to your urethra.

- Avoid wearing tight pants.

- Drinking four or more glasses of unsweetened cranberry juice, mixed with nonchlorinated water, causes the urine to be more acidic. Acidic urine helps prevent UTI's. If you feel an infection coming on, begin drinking cranberry juice and the herbs listed below, follow dietary recommendations, and rest. Incorporating the various preventive measures into your daily life will greatly reduce your need for drugs.

- Avoid air-conditioned rooms if possible and avoid sitting in cold or damp areas. These environments weaken the kidneys, making a person more susceptible to infection.

Dietary Support

Eat a light diet of steamed, dark green leafy vegetables, brown rice, and other whole grains. After the acute symptoms have subsided, begin adding a small amount of adzuki beans, black soy beans, or black beans with garlic and sea vegetables into your diet. These beans strengthen the kidneys and immune system. (Too much protein stresses the kidneys. Obtain your protein sources from vegetables.) Avoid ingesting cold foods and beverages as they wear out the kidneys. In the summertime you can eat watermelon that is room temperature for cleansing the kidneys. A healing diet will help prevent recurring infections.

Supplements

Vitamin C—500 mg every hour until acute symptoms subside. Then take 1000–2000 mg, two to three times daily

Beta-carotene—50,000 IU, twice daily

Zinc—15 mg daily

Organic flax-seed oil—mix 2–3 teaspoons, twice a day, with grains, steamed vegetables, or soup

Herbal Support

A combination of the following herbs in tea or tincture form works well at clearing up a urinary tract infection. They work quickly if you begin using them as soon as you feel an infection coming on or if you have been diagnosed with a UTI. When using tinctures, put the drops in hot water and let sit five minutes, allowing the alcohol to evaporate.

Echinacea root—3 parts

Corn silk—1 part

Pipsissewa—1 part

Cleavers—2 parts

Usnea lichen (usnea is not soluble in water—use in tincture form)—2 parts

Bearberry, also called uva ursi (pregnant women avoid)—2 parts

Dose and Use: To make tea, place 1 tablespoon of echinacea root into 1 quart of water and simmer for thirty minutes. Add 1–2 teaspoons of the other herbs and steep, covered, for ten to fifteen minutes. Drink ½ cup of tea, or take 20–40 drops of tincture, every hour until the acute symptoms subside. Then continue drinking 3–5 cups of tea, or taking the tincture three to five times per day, for another ten days to ensure the infection is gone. Rest as much as possible.

If blood is present in your urine add yarrow flowers and/or horsetail into the above formula along with seeking appropriate help. If you are experiencing strong cramping add crampbark to the above herbs.

For women who have recurring UTI's, follow the suggestions listed above, along with taking equal parts of couchgrass rhizomes (a despised weed in most gardens, commonly called quack grass or witch grass by farmers) yarrow flowers, and marshmallow leaf as a tea or tincture, three to four times a week to help strengthen and nourish urinary tract tissue. Homeopathic constitutional treatment works well for both chronic and acute UTI's.

A full body bath can feel relaxing and relieve pain during an infection.

A sitz bath improves circulation in the pelvic area. Fill a plastic tub with warm water that comes up to your navel. Be warm before doing a sitz bath—take a warm shower or bath beforehand. Sit in the tub and hang your feet over the side.

A chronic urinary tract infection may be a sign of a deeper problem. Pelvic congestion, chronic constipation, heavy or painful

menstruation, exhaustion, bloatedness, and gastrointestinal problems may accompany chronic UTI's. All these problems need to be
addressed with your health care provider.

LESBIAN HEALTH

There are several reasons why I have included a section on lesbian
health in this book. First, I have not seen lesbian health issues
directly addressed in other women's herb books. As a lesbian, I see
a need for women's health books to be inclusive in their language
and orientation. I feel frustrated, alienated, and invisible when the
prevailing tone, attitude, and information is directed at women in
relationships with men. Second, I have included specific lesbian
health concerns throughout the book as a way to continue to edu-
cate myself, other lesbians, bisexual women, heterosexual women,
and health care providers. I have yet to find many clinical health
studies specific to lesbian or bisexual women. There may be more,
but my search certainly proved how unimportant lesbian health is
to the medical community. I also found little written information on
lesbians and sexually transmitted diseases other than a few pamphlets on lesbians and HIV. Third, I wanted to speak directly to
how the oppressive and negative attitudes toward lesbians, prevalent in the United States, affect our self-esteem, sense of safety, and
overall health.

I wish to acknowledge bisexual women as a group that sometimes feels alienated by both lesbians and heterosexual women.
Throughout this book when I speak on lesbian health issues I am
also including bisexual women.

While I was writing this book I went to the first lesbian health
conference held in Maine. One of the areas discussed was the need
for a resource list of health care providers in Maine who are educated, sensitive, and respectful of lesbians and their health needs. I
suspect this is a need in most places around the country, especially
in rural areas. Many lesbians do not receive good quality health care
or the kind of care they specifically need because the medical profession seems to operate under the assumption that all women are
heterosexual. There are studies that show that most health care
providers receive little or no training on lesbian health issues. Many

are openly homophobic, some are verbally or physically abusive toward lesbians, and some even suggest lesbians seek out psychiatric care to correct their "problem." Many ask insensitive questions and assume that because you are a woman you have sex with men and need birth control. Lesbians sometimes do not get the appropriate diagnosis or medical treatment because they do not feel safe enough to disclose their sexuality.

Because health insurance plans are expensive and do not recognize a lesbian's partner, during a medical emergency a lesbian's partner has no legal power to sign papers unless she has obtained power of attorney beforehand. Even with power of attorney, hospital visitations, especially entering the intensive care unit, can be difficult or impossible for the lesbian partner.

Pregnancy, adoption, and parenting are big areas of concern for some lesbians. Fertility issues, questions about insemination, finding an adoption agency that will work with lesbians, receiving respectful and supportive care throughout the pregnancy and birth, finding a school that is open and respectful to lesbian mothers and their children, getting support about parenting issues, and losing custody of children because of being lesbian are all situations that present various difficulties.

Living in a society that outwardly discriminates against lesbians and gay men is emotionally and mentally exhausting and this added stress takes its toll on the body in different ways. To continually hear negative comments about lesbians (or to be ignored) in the workplace, by religious organizations, government and medical institutions, and local community members is hurtful. Issues concerning coming out—who is it safe to come out to, what will friends and/or family members think or say, fear of losing one's job or being refused housing—are challenging situations for many lesbians.

As with any so-called minority group, lesbians also come from diverse ethnic, religious, and class backgrounds, various age groups and levels of education, and have differences in physical abilities. Some are single, some have one sexual partner, and some have many lovers. Some lesbians have never had a sexual relationship with a man, some are celibate, and some have relationships with both women and men. Some lesbians call themselves feminists and some do not. Some consider themselves to be separatists. Some lesbians have been battered by men and some by women. Some are from rural areas and others are from urban centers. Lesbians' experiences are far reaching and each woman's life story affects her self-esteem and overall health.

The need for more medical information concerning health issues specific to lesbians and more informed health care providers, both mainstream and holistic, is obvious. Medical people usually know little about how women transmit infections to each other, rarely know the answers to how lesbian lovemaking may relate to a specific gynecological problem, or which dis-eases are more prevalent among lesbians. Chapter 8 addresses vaginitis and how women can pass various vaginal infections to each other. The HIV virus can be passed between women lovers, and honest communication about past and/or present lovers is essential to ensure the virus is not spread. Herpes and the human papilloma virus can also be spread between women. Though sexually transmitted diseases are less often passed between women lovers, they can be and they are. Health pamphlets that specifically address the health concerns of lesbians are desperately needed in all health care centers, schools, clinics, and hospitals along with respectful health protocols for health care providers working with women.

Loving another person, whichever sex, is worthy of celebration. As we all come to better understand both the wonderful and challenging things in each other's lives, we will have more information with which to help end the various oppressions different groups of women and men face.

> During the process of bringing about change in our society, lesbians need to keep in mind that we've got to take care of, and bring about change in, ourselves, our sisters, and our families— while at the same time confronting the larger issues that are making us sick. We need to develop the balance between being strong enough to fight social injustices and lesbian oppression, and gentle enough to nurture our bodies, our minds, and each other.[6]

10

As We Grow Older

Together we are building a new road to aging, and at the same time that road is building us. Young women have as great a stake in our efforts as older women do, for their turn is coming. . . . When we finally bridge the generation gap, women will be a magnificent force for positive change in society.[1]

—OURSELVES, GROWING OLDER

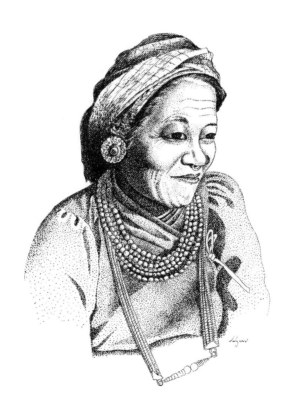

Aging is a journey we are all experiencing. The issues vary and change the older we grow. For example, racial, economic, and social factors affect the quality and length of a woman's life. These factors differ from country to country and within a country.

Middle-aged and elderly women are seen and responded to differently, depending on cultural views and customs. At one time, older women were highly respected and held decision-making positions in many traditional cultures. Western society, however, generally regards women beyond childbearing years as worthless and needy. Negative images are reinforced by the media and the pharmaceutical industry and these often influence how we feel about ourselves. As women continue to speak and write about growing older, these denigrating attitudes will change.

New frontiers open as we grow older. Some offer challenges and others we welcome without hesitation. Menopause can be a difficult time for some women and an easy transition for others. Events like children leaving home, reentering school, elderly parents needing care, illness and death of family members, primary relationships changing or ending, sexuality issues arising, job changes, and decreases in physical energy add new dimensions to growing older. Some women have shared with me that they feel a spiritual aspect to their aging; a graceful acceptance of themselves, periods of heightened creativity and dreams, a quiet, inward strength developing, and a shift into deeper realms within their psyches. Aging is a journey we are all experiencing. The more we share our stories with each other the less likely we are to feel isolated and scared.

MENOPAUSE

In 1987 I was driving to a conference on menopause to teach a workshop on herbs. When I realized I had started my period early I pulled into a small grocery store to buy some pads. My old Volvo would not start up again. I ran across the street to a gas station to call home and noticed a woman pull up in an old Volkswagen bug. I asked if she was headed near Bangor and could she give me a ride. She said yes. I ran back to my car to get my slides and a basket full of herbs. She shook her head when she saw my basket and asked what on earth was I up to. I told her I was teaching about herbs for menopause at a conference. She looked at me and started laughing and said, "Now honey, what does a girl your age know about menopause?" I smiled and nodded my head in agreement. She proceeded to tell me stories about her life, including her menopause time, which for her was an easy transition.

I have yet to begin menopause and am grateful for the many opportunities I have had to listen to women's menopause stories at conferences and in smaller circles. Recently I was asked to participate as the herbalist with four other women (a woman experiencing menopause, a medical doctor, a nutritionist, and a therapist) on a panel about menopause. More than one hundred women gathered for two and a half hours on an evening that also happened to be a full moon. The energy in the room was very charged. The women sat on the edges of their seats, listening attentively to the information and stories being shared and asking poignant questions. We could have continued on for half the night. I felt excited to be in a room full of women eager to be more knowledgeable about their bodies.

Menopause is a transition period that lasts from several months up to a few years. It is the end of fertility only, not the end of sexuality or creativity. A silence still surrounds menopause, similar to the silence around menstruation. Misinformation about this passage instills fear in many women as they enter their forties and begin to think about menopause. Books such as *Ourselves, Growing Older* by the Boston Women's Health Collective and women's support groups offer women the chance to read and exchange correct information and receive emotional and spiritual support. The highest number of women ever to reach menopause on our planet is occurring now because women are living longer. As more women enter this time of change valuing their bodies, viewing menopause as an opportunity for new growth, and embracing their inner wisdom, the negative and false images of menopause will fade.

Menopause commonly begins for women during their mid to late forties. Changes in the amount of blood flow, how often and how long periods last, hot flashes, vaginal dryness, and varying emotional states are some common signs of menopause. Other body symptoms may occur, such as: depression, memory loss, heart palpitations, nausea, insomnia, anxiety, circulatory problems, sore breasts, water retention, dry eyes or skin, a decrease in sexual energy, hypoglycemia, and congestion of the lower abdomen. The lack of correct and supportive literature and negative societal attitudes about the physiological and emotional changes of this natural phase of our life's cycle leave many women totally disconnected from their body's process, drugged, or pretending menopause is not happening.

The whole process, from the first signs of menopause until menstruation finally stops and one's body adjusts to the hormonal changes, is menopause. During this time the ovaries secrete less and less estrogen and progesterone. Estrogen levels may drop suddenly for some women and gradually for others. Sometimes estrogen levels shift radically, causing the menstrual flow to be heavier or lighter for some months and not present at all other months. The hormonal fluctuations that change the regularity of one's menstrual cycle may last for several months or years. Other variables come into play, such as cultural views of menopause, a woman's health history, access to nutritional food, economic status, and adrenal stress.

The adrenal glands play a central role in our health, especially as we move into and beyond menopause. They help our bodies deal with various kinds of stresses and play a role in maintaining our resistance to dis-ease. As our ovaries begin to secrete less and less estrogen, the adrenals take over this job. The adrenals convert a secretion called androstenadione into estrone in our blood and body fat. Exercising regularly and having some fat on our bones supports this transition. The media's portrayal of thin as the "right" way for women to be is detrimental to women on many levels, particularly as we approach menopause. It is to our advantage to have some fat on us to help maintain estrogen levels in our body.

Many of us have overworked adrenals due to stressful lifestyles and poor diets even before we reach menopause. Fatigue, depression, irritability, and nervous system dis-eases are signs of overworked adrenal glands. Dietary changes, herbs, and lifestyle changes help strengthen the adrenal glands for women during their twenties, thirties, and forties and will help the menopause transition be smoother. Regular weight-bearing exercise is the other crucial area for younger women to address before reaching menopause because it helps maintain bone density, thus helping to prevent osteoporosis after menopause.

Those of us who have grown up in Western cultures are often challenged with the need to be producing—basically to be super-women—and we overwork all the time, to feel worthwhile or to survive financially. This treadmill is difficult to get off. We desperately need to rewrite the script. Our energy shifts from being outwardly productive and active to being more inwardly focused and creative as we approach, and move beyond, menopause.

As we grow older we do not have the same energy reserves to draw upon as when we were twenty. It is time for us to rearrange our priorities so we are doing things that we enjoy instead of doing things we dislike and that drain us of our creative energy and vital life force. If we continue to overwork, taking no time to be still and quiet each day, our bodies and spirits weaken more quickly.

This is the time of life for women to fully embrace their creative and spiritual selves. We have accumulated many life experiences by the time we reach menopause. By moving more deeply into our inner selves we can incorporate what we have learned into our psyches and the wisdom that comes with age will grace us. The image of the crone, a woman who is honoring her inner voice and living life how she chooses, is a powerful one to visualize at this time for oneself and for all aging women.

NUTRITIONAL SUPPORT

A balanced diet, low in fat, caffeine, sugar, salt, white flour, and alcohol and high in mineral- and vitamin-rich foods, supports the body's hormonal changes and the adrenal glands and is essential in preventing osteoporosis and heart disease. Whole grains, dark leafy green vegetables, sea vegetables, moderate protein from legumes, nuts, seeds, and seasonal fruit are the foundational foods for a balanced diet. Regular exercise, love, and adequate rest and relaxation are also important aspects of a healthy lifestyle that I hope someday all women will experience.

Nicotine and alcohol can be difficult for many women to eliminate completely and it is important to be aware of how they adversely affect the body. Nicotine poisons the ovaries, interfering with estrogen production as well as various adrenal functions. Alcohol consumption stresses the adrenal glands, liver, gastrointestinal tract, and the immune system. Regular use of alcohol also suppresses ovarian function.

Coffee, black tea, and a high intake of dairy products leach calcium out of the blood. Milk is too high in phosphorus and upsets the calcium/phosphorus balance in the blood. Calcium is leached out of the blood in order to rebalance the blood's calcium/phosphorus levels.

SUPPLEMENTS

- Vitamin E–400 IU, taken twice daily with meals. Buy d-alpha and mixed tocopherol rather than dl-alpha as it is better quality.

  Vitamin E nourishes the reproductive and cardiovascular systems of the body when taken on a daily basis. It helps to diminish hot flashes, vaginal dryness, itching, and muscle cramps. It is a fat soluble vitamin and needs to be taken with meals.

  Note: For women with high blood pressure, diabetes, and heart problems, keep your intake to 50–100 IU per day.
- Vitamin D–350–400 IU daily. (Women need a bit more vitamin D as we age; sixty and older use 400–800 IU daily.)
- Vitamin C–2000 mg per day, or more if needed
- Beta-carotene–25,000 IU, twice daily
- Iron–Iron is essential for ensuring that the blood is properly oxygenated. The body feels tired and run down if iron levels are low. Refer to chapter 6 for iron-rich herbs and food.
- Calcium and Magnesium–Adequate calcium and magnesium intake is crucial for strong bones. Calcium needs the presence of magnesium in order to be absorbed. Calcium and magnesium compete for the same receptor sites in the stomach for absorption, so it is essential they be taken together in the right proportions.

You can eat calcium- and magnesium-rich foods and take supplements, but unless your stomach lining is producing adequate levels of hydrochloric acid (HCl) your body will not absorb calcium or other nutrients from food. HCl begins to lower as we age, and 40 percent of postmenopausal women have low HCl levels and are not absorbing calcium.[2]

It is important for premenopausal and postmenopausal women to have enough HCl for calcium absorption. To insure HCl production at the beginning of each meal take digestive bitter herbs such as blessed thistle, burdock root, and gentian root (described in chapter 5), 1–2 tablespoons of freshly squeezed lemon juice in a cup of water, or 2 tablespoons of apple cider vinegar or rice vinegar in a cup of water. AVOID all antacid pills as they lower HCl levels.

Calcium (Ca) citrate and magnesium (Mg) citrate are the most easily absorbed forms of calcium and magnesium in supplement form. Avoid calcium made from oyster shells and dolomite. Mary Lynn Garner, N.D., recommends 800–1000 mg of calcium and 400–750 mg of magnesium be taken twice daily, at breakfast and just before bedtime.

- Bioflavanoids—Foods and herbs high in bioflavanoids such as blueberries, blackberries, and hawthorn berries improve the integrity of the collagen matrix, which keeps joints and connective tissue strong and healthy and reduces inflamed joints. These foods are safe and nourishing to eat on a regular basis, even long before menopause.

My favorite way to take hawthorn berries is in a concentrated paste form that requires several gallons of berries cooked at a very low temperature. Hawthorn berry paste can be found in some health food stores or ordered through Avena Botanicals.

Besides being rich in bioflavanoids, hawthorn berries taken with the flowers and leaves is a cardiovascular tonic. Research done in Europe has proven the safety and effectiveness of the whole herb when taken over several months on a daily basis. Hawthorn helps to restore cardiovascular tone, improves coronary circulation, nourishes the cells of the cardiac muscle, normalizes blood pressure (taken with other herbs such as linden flowers, garlic, parsley, and skullcap) reduces the possibility of angina attacks by dilating the coronary arteries, and aids in the healing process of back injuries, hemorrhoids, and varicosities. Hawthorn is a safe herb for a person who has experienced a heart attack or stroke, or whose family has a history of heart disease, to add into their health plan. It is food for the heart and in my opinion a food we would all benefit from taking on a daily basis.

- Essential fatty acids–Essential fatty acids are important for many reasons. They help maintain the health of the cell membranes of all the body's cells, help the body process prostaglandins type I and III, and keep the vagina and skin from becoming overly dry. Prostaglandins are hormonelike chemicals that regulate blood pressure and play an important role in lowering the risk of heart disease. Prostaglandins I and III have been shown to reduce PMS symptoms and menstrual cramps and strengthen the immune system.

Fresh flax-seed oil is an essential fatty acid that contains both linoleic (Omega-6) and linolenic acids (Omega-3). This oil has a light buttery flavor and is a delicious addition to steamed vegetables or cooked grains. Good quality, organic flax-seed oil is now available in most health food stores. It must be stored in the refrigerator and used up within six weeks. Two teaspoons, taken twice daily, is the recommended dose for adults. Menopausal women may need 2–3 tablespoons daily along with vitamin E to reduce vaginal dryness and dry skin and hair.

Mineral-Rich Tea

The green weeds and nourishing herbs are strong allies as we grow older. They offer vitamins and minerals and are infused with a vibrant life force that supports our journey. Remember the consistency with which herbs are taken is important for truly benefiting the body in an ongoing way. The following herbs are rich in various minerals and vitamins.

Alfalfa—1 part

Borage leaf—2 parts

Chamomile—1 part

Hawthorn flowers and berries—1 part

Horsetail—1 part

Nettle leaf—1 part

Oatstraw—2 parts

Raspberry leaves—1 part

Red clover—2 parts

Violet leaves and flowers—1 part

Dose and Use: Let 2–3 teaspoons of herbs steep in a cup of hot steaming water, covered, for ten to fifteen minutes. Drink 1–3 cups per day, warm or cool.

Adrenal Support Tincture

The following herbs strengthen the adrenal glands and stabilize hormonal function. This formula gives extra nutrition to all glands in the body, especially the adrenals, improves overall energy and physical endurance, and stimulates the body's vital life force.

Siberian ginseng root—2 parts

Saw palmetto berries—1 part

Schizandra berries—1 part

Prickly ash bark—1 part

Licorice root—¼ part

Dose and Use: Take as a tincture, 25–50 drops, two to three times daily, between meals. Most effective when used consistently over several months.

General Menopause Tonic

The following herbs help regulate hormonal changes and strengthen the nervous system. This formula offers general support to a woman experiencing menopause. Herbs that help ease specific menopausal symptoms such as hot flashes or vaginal dryness are included further on in this chapter.

Vitex berries—3 parts

Motherwort—2 parts

Fresh milky wild oat seed—2 parts

Dong Quai root—1 part

Wild yam root—1 part

False unicorn root—1 part

Licorice root—¼ part

Dose and Use: Take as a tincture, 25–50 drops, two to three times per day, five to six days a week. Can be used over several months.

Root Tea

Root teas help to ground and center us. The following herbs support the changing hormones, nourish the blood, give strength to the immune system, and increase physical energy and well-being.

Astragalus root—2 parts

Burdock root—1 part

Codonopsis root—1 part

Cinnamon bark—1 part

Dong Quai root—1 part

Licorice root—1 part

Rehmannia (cooked)—2 parts

Vitex berries—2 parts

Dose and Use: Mix the herbs together and measure ¼–½ cup into a glass or enamel pot. Pour 2–3 quarts of water over the herbs and simmer, covered, for 30–40 minutes. Drink 1–2 cups per day, three to five times a week. You can pour more water over the roots and simmer again. The flavor will be a little weaker the second time around. If you have a tendency to feel cold, add a pinch of dried ginger to the tea to help improve circulation.

American Ginseng

American ginseng is another root to consider during menopause. I am fortunate to have had the oppurtunity to go "seng" hunting with my friend Doug Elliot in the North Carolina mountains one fall. American ginseng is a beautiful plant and in the fall the red berries are what a digger looks for.

Unfortunately, wild American ginseng has been overharvested in this country and in some places, like Maine, there are very few plants left. On the up side there are some people beginning to organically cultivate American ginseng in the United States.

When taken consistently over several weeks or months, ginseng slowly rebuilds and restores the body's overall energy and vitality and helps counteract stress and fatigue, nourishes the hormonal system, eases hot flashes, and evens out feelings of emotional instability.

Some women like taking American ginseng while others do not like the stimulation their bodies feel when they take it. Start out with smaller doses of tincture, 5–10 drops, or ¼ or ½ cup of tea, and see how your body responds. If you feel overstimulated then discontinue use.

Note: Siberian ginseng and American ginseng are completely different plants. A good quality Siberian ginseng tincture can also be taken daily by any age person over many months to increase physical energy and endurance and help the body be better able to cope with stress. You could experiment with each ginseng and see which one you prefer. Be sure to know where either of these roots come from.

HOT FLASHES

Women's experiences of hot flashes vary as to when and how often they occur, how long they last, and for how many years. Heart palpitations and feelings of anxiety or nausea accompany hot flashes for some women, while other women are awakened during the night drenched in sweat; still others experience only a warm sensation that passes easily. When a hot flash occurs, blood vessels dilate and the blood flow to the skin increases. The internal body temperature actually drops while the skin temperature increases four to eight degrees. Sweating and increased blood flow to the skin is the body's mechanism for eliminating heat from the body. Hot flashes usually end when the body adjusts to lower levels of estrogen.

Hot flashes can be stronger and more frequent in women whose ovaries have been removed before they reached menopause, especially during the first six months following surgery. When the ovaries are removed surgically before menopause, the estrogen levels drop immediately. Even if a woman has her ovaries removed after menopause she will often experience hot flashes.

Along with the physiological explanations of hot flashes come various theories about the insights women may glean from them. Some women call them power surges, the body's releasing of energy. When you can, give yourself some space to explore your inner journey. What messages from your depths may be rising forth at this time in your life?

❀

Wise Woman Tea

This tea helps to ease hot flashes, night sweats, and anxiety.

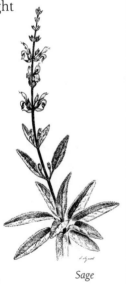

Sage

Sage—2 parts

Motherwort—1 part

Hawthorn flowers, leaves, and berries—
1 part

Alfalfa—3 parts

Oatstraw—1 part

Fenugreek seed—1 part

Fennel seed—2 parts

Licorice root—½ part

Dose and Use: Place 5–6 tablespoons in a glass pot or jar, pour a quart of hot steaming water over the herbs, and let steep, covered, for fifteen to twenty minutes. Drink 3–4 cups per day.

If you find yourself waking up drenched with sweat or sweating more than is comfortable during the day, drink 1–3 cups of warm sage tea (*Salvia officinalis*) throughout the day. This sage is easy to grow in the garden. It is a perennial, yet after four or five years you may want to take cuttings from your original plant when it gets woody and begins to die back or start new plants from seed. Sage tea is a nice addition to your bath and a soothing and antiseptic tea for easing a sore throat and gargling with. Dried sage may be placed in a dream pillow to help bring up the inner wisdom we all carry deep inside, and can be burned in your home and work environment to clear the air.

Wise Woman Tincture

This tincture can be used alone or in conjunction with the above tea and the General Menopause Tonic to lessen the uncomfortable symptoms of hot flashes.

Blessed thistle—1 part

False unicorn root—1 part

Motherwort—3 parts

Vitex berries—2 parts

Wild yam root—2 parts

Dose and Use: Take 30–50 drops, two to three times per day, over several weeks or months.

MOOD SWINGS

Many menopausal women have been unjustly targeted as irrational and overly emotional, especially if they begin to express deeply buried rage or the truth that they have previously kept quiet about so as not to "rock the boat" within their families or workplaces. Some women feel as if their lives are falling apart; things that they once thought were secure begin to change, including partnerships, jobs, and their health. More than ever, women need to be listened to well by people who support them and have an understanding and respect for the difficulties and opportunities that present themselves during menopause.

Herbs and flower essences can be helpful allies from the plant world during times of tremendous change. We can also get so caught up in using herbs that we do not give ourselves space to feel whatever feelings are emerging. Keep listening to the wise woman within you and she will guide you.

Nervine Tincture

The following herbs nourish and strengthen the nervous system and ease nervous tension, anxiety, mental and emotional exhaustion, debility, and restlessness.

Fresh, milky oats—2 parts

Schizandra berries—1 part

Polygala—1 part

Fresh lemon balm—2 parts

Rosemary—1 part

Lavender—1 part

Dose and Use: As a tincture, take 20–40 drops, three to four times per day over one to four months.

Nervine Tea

The following herbs are soothing and calming to the spirit and body. Drink a cup of tea whenever you want.

Lemon balm—2 parts

Linden blossom—1 part

Lemon verbena—2 parts

Lavender—1 part

Oatstraw—1 part

Dose and Use: Pour a cup of hot steaming water over 2–3 teaspoons of herbs. Steep, covered, for five to ten minutes and drink warm.

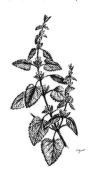

Lemon Balm

A warm bath with a few drops of the essential oils of lemon balm, marjoram, and mugwort is soothing and relaxing. You can also make a quart of tea with these three herbs by placing 1–2 table-spoons of each herb into a glass quart jar and covering with hot steaming water. Steep, covered, for fifteen to thirty minutes. Strain and add into the bathwater.

DRY EYES AND MOUTH

Some women find their eyes and/or mouth become dryer during menopause. Calendula flowers are my favorite herb to use for this condition. Make a strong tea from fresh or dried calendula blossoms. Strain the tea and rinse your mouth and/or eyes as often as you need. Drinking calendula and oatstraw tea more regularly may also help. If you have fresh chickweed growing in your garden you can add that into your eye- and mouthwash and into your tea.

INSOMNIA

I have heard many women talk about being unable to sleep in the same way they are accustomed to when they go through menopause. When you can sleep, let yourself sleep. Take any opportunity you can to nap when your body seems ready to fall asleep. Easier said than done for most of us. Feeling deprived of a sound sleep for days on end is not only physically but also emotionally exhausting.

During transition times our body's old ways of doing things

can change. We are being asked by our deep unconscious to rearrange our outward life to meet our inward needs. Keeping a dream journal, writing, painting, dancing, meditating, and singing are some ways to express your inward journey and allow your creativity to flow freely. Other methods to consider may include deep relaxation techniques, body work, prayer, and psychotherapy.

Sleep Tea

If you are unable to sleep because your nervous system and mind feel overactive, the following tea can be taken every day to help nourish nerves and calm the body.

Oatstraw—2 parts
Lemon balm—2 parts
Linden—2 parts
Skullcap—1 part
Chamomile—1 part
Lavender—1 part
Blue vervain—1 part

Dose and Use: Steep 1–2 tablespoons of herbs in a cup of hot steaming water, covered, for five to fifteen minutes. Drink warm.

Sleep Tincture

Hops—1 part
Skullcap—1 part
Motherwort—1 part
Passion flower—1 part

St. Johnswort—1 part

Valerian root—2 parts

Dose and Use: Take 25–50 drops of tincture one-half hour before bedtime and take again if you awaken in the night and you want to sleep more. Also include the General Menopause Tonic in your daily health plan.

VAGINAL CHANGES

The mucous membrane lining of the vagina becomes thinner and holds less moisture as we age. This thinning is the result of less estrogen being produced in the ovaries. For some women the thinning feels extremely uncomfortable if the vagina becomes dry or inflamed. Doctors commonly prescribe estrogen creams and pills to ease this condition.

Fortunately, a nourishing diet, drinking three to four glasses of clean water a day, added moisture in your home, vitamin E capsules or suppositories inserted into the vagina, taking the General Menopause Tonic and Adrenal Support Tincture listed above, and doing Kegel exercises releases discomforts associated with thinning vaginal membranes. Kegal exercises are the tightening and releasing of the pubococcygeus (PC) muscle, which is the muscle that stops urination and tightens the anus, several times a day. Work up to 25–50 per day within the first few weeks and continue increasing up to 200 per day. Orgasms can also help relieve the shrinking and thinning discomforts.

An herb oil or salve made from herbs such as calendula flowers, plantain, St. Johnswort flowers, and comfrey root and leaves relieves vaginal itching, dryness, inflammation, and soreness. Apply as often as needed on the labia and inside the vagina. Lubricate the vagina with an herb oil, salve, or vitamin E oil before engaging in any sexual interaction.

Vitamin E capsules or suppositories inserted into the vagina will also heal an inflamed or irritated vaginal lining and lessen vaginal dryness. Use six nights a week for several weeks if condition is severe.

Osteoporosis and Hormone Replacement Therapy

Osteoporosis is an important women's health issue in the Western world and ten times as many women as men are affected. More than one million bone fractures occur each year, usually starting with wrist fractures and spinal fractures in women in their fifties and moving into hip fractures as women reach their sixties and seventies.

Bone density in women peaks at about age thirty-five and slowly begins to decrease over time. Regular weight-bearing exercise and good nutrition are two of the most important factors for women to incorporate into their lives as early as possible for preventing osteoporosis.

Proper calcium intake is important, but not the only nutritional factor to consider when building and maintaining strong bones. There are many factors that interfere with the exchange of calcium between the blood and bones, including a diet high in protein and fat, inability of the gastrointestinal tract to absorb calcium, a vitamin D deficiency, and hormonal fluctuations.

A high protein diet, the norm in Western countries, has been medically shown to have a weakening effect on the skeletal structure. High protein and fat inhibit calcium absorption. Dairy food, though stressed by the American Dairy Council as the essential food for getting calcium, is not at all the appropriate food for receiving adequate levels of calcium. Dairy foods do not have the proper calcium/phosphorus ratio for absorption, which is two to one. Dairy food contains a ratio of one to one. Other things that deplete the body of calcium include carbonated drinks, caffeine, high salt intake, high sugar diets, and stress. Stress can double the urinary excretion of calcium from the body.[3]

Certain factors do make women more at risk for osteoporosis. These include being fair skinned, thin, and short; coming from a Northern European bloodline; having had a teenage pregnancy or not having birthed children; having a lactose intolerance; or having a family history of osteoporosis. Other situations that put us at risk besides the dietary concerns and lack of regular exercise discussed above include smoking, high alcohol intake, extensive fasting or dieting, anorexia, diabetes, chronic diarrhea, kidney or liver disease, removal of the ovaries, onset of menopause before age forty, and specific prescription and over-the-counter drugs.

The media and medical system lead the public to believe that low estrogen levels are a leading cause of osteoporosis and therefore hormone replacement therapy (HRT) must be given to all menopausal women. Fortunately, there are some wise doctors out there working with women who are at risk or who already have osteoporosis, and reversals in the condition are occurring with regular, weight-bearing exercise, twenty minutes or one-half hour daily, three times per week; a low fat and low protein diet; adequate vitamin and mineral supplementation, and the use of low doses of estrogen and pro-gest cream applied topically.[4] Women who cannot take estrogen may find using pro-gest cream (available in women's health clinics and from health care providers) and certain herbs to be helpful.

Remember when debating whether to use a hormone replacement therapy that menopause is a natural part of our body's cycle. Most of the uncomfortable symptoms that come on with menopause do not last forever. Many doctors view this passage as a disease and insist that women must take drugs. Menopause is not a disease. It is a powerful passage into the next phase of life. Western culture has a phobia about aging and dying that often gets associated with the menopause time. Wrinkles and the shifting of our energy are natural progressions of aging that we need to acknowledge and not inhibit with unnecessary drugs.

There is a place for HRT, but it is overprescribed today and should not be used by women who have uterine fibroids, endometriosis, liver or gallbladder diseases, or depression, or by women at risk for uterine or breast cancer. It is also important to note that women with a Native American background are at higher risk for gallbladder disease and should also avoid hormone replacement.[5]

The lack of money put toward research on women's health issues leaves us with many unanswered questions about the long-term safety of HRT. Each woman must make her own health care choices based on what she feels best about. For me, I always come back to believing in myself, in my intelligence, in my intuition, in Earth's healing energy, and in the caregivers I seek out for guidance.

HERBAL SUPPORT

There are women who have successfully reduced or eliminated their intake of estrogen over six months to a year with the help of herbs. Do so very gradually, paying close attention to how you feel. If uncomfortable symptoms arise, stay with the dosage of hormones that works for you for a while and then begin the reduction process again. Staying in contact with a knowledgeable herbalist or health care provider can be helpful. Besides following the guidelines previously discussed, use the Adrenal Support Tincture, Mineral-Rich Tea, and vitamin supplementation in conjunction with the following tincture.

> Fresh milky oats—1 part
>
> Blessed thistle—1 part
>
> Dong Quai root—2 parts
>
> False unicorn root—2 parts
>
> Licorice root—2 parts
>
> Sarsaparilla root—2 parts
>
> Wild yam root—3 parts
>
> Vitex berries—2 parts

Dose and Use: Take 30–50 drops of tincture, three to four times per day, five to six days a week, over several months.

Note: For women concerned about intake of the strongly estrogenic herbs, herbalist Amanda McQuade Crawford suggests avoiding intake of black cohosh and Dong Quai.

AGING GRACEFULLY

A few years back I taught a day-long workshop on women's health at a small college. Thirty women of various ages attended. At the end of the day, a woman approached me and said the workshop was good, but what about the issues of women beyond menopause. As I asked her what she would recommend be included in future workshops, I remembered the following statement written by Barbara MacDonald, who coauthored *Look Me In the Eyes* with Cynthia Rich:

If an old woman talks about arthritis or cataracts, don't think old women are constantly complaining. We are just trying to get a word in edgewise while you talk about abortions, contraception, premenstrual syndrome, toxic shock, or turkey basters.[5]

So what about life beyond menopause? Finally women are talking about menstruation and menopause more openly than ten years ago, but what about older women's issues? Yes, we are beginning to see more books and organizations addressing the numerous oppressions aging women face every day. Yet what will it take for Western society to seriously confront ageism, to stop exploiting aging people, either placing them on pedestals and seeing them only as our teachers, or leaving them to die alone in nursing homes or apartments? The Women's Health Movement and various other feminist movements have made important steps forward in improving the lives of women and children. Yet for us all to benefit we need to fully understand ageism, how each of us has internalized false and hurtful attitudes toward aging women, and how directly linked the roots of ageism are to oppressive patriarchal values.

Aging women's issues are numerous and as complex and as varied as women are. Refer to the resource section for titles on specific topics. At this point in my life I lack the experience to write a whole chapter on herbs for aging women. Included are a few formulas that have benefited different women. For a more thorough herbal I recommend *An Elder's Herbal*, by David Hoffman.

Daily Tonic

The following herbs help to increase vitality and resiliancy, keep the fire of life shining in one's eyes, help prevent memory loss, and nourish the nervous system.

Orange peel—1 part

Hawthorn flowers, leaves, and berries—2 parts

Ginkgo leaves—2 parts

Siberian ginseng root—2 parts

Sacred basil flowers and leaves—1 part

Fresh milky oat seed—1 part

Use and Dose: Take as a tincture, 15–25 drops, two to three times per day over several months.

Flower Tea

One of my favorite children's books is called *Wildflower Tea*, by Ethel Pochocki. I was inspired to create my own flower tea after reading this story. The following flowers happen to be my favorites. Use whatever flowers and proportions you prefer. A glass jar with all these herbs combined together looks like a beautiful garden.

Sacred basil flowers and leaves

Calendula flowers

Lemon balm

Linden flowers

Rose petals

Anise-hyssop

Dose and Use: Pour 1 cup of hot steaming water over 2–3 tablespoons of herbs and steep five to ten minutes, covered, and drink warm or cool.

Circulation Tonic

A nourishing formula for nonacute and long-term heart-related conditions. These herbs improve overall circulation, thus helping to warm the body if it is cold, tone heart muscle, circulate blood and oxygen to the brain, and help resolve nervous conditions related to the vascular system. Seek appropriate health care for serious heart conditions or if you wish to use herbs in conjunction with heart medications.

Hawthorn berries, leaves, and flowers—2 parts
Ginkgo leaves—3 parts
Motherwort—1 part
Codonopsis root—1 part
Prickly ash bark—1 part

Dose and Use: As a tincture, take 20–40 drops, two to three times per day, four to five times a week.

Cataract Eye Wash

A daily eye wash with dusty miller (*Cineraria maritima*) and eyebright may be of help in the early stages of cataracts. Make a strong tea combining equal parts of these herbs, 2 tablespoons steeped, covered, in 1 cup of boiled water. Let steep four to eight hours. Strain and use an eye cup. Store leftover tea in the refrigerator up to four days. Rinse eyes with tea that is room temperature.

Cataract Surgery Support Herbs

Begin taking a good quality Siberian ginseng tincture at least two to four weeks before surgery, twice a day, to support the body's response to the stress of surgery along with drinking nettle, red clover, and calendula tea. Continue taking the tincture and tea for several months after, one to two times a day. Take homeopathic arnica, 30c, twice daily the day before, the day of, and the day after surgery to ease shock, trauma, and bruising. Consult a trained homeopath if you want a specific remedy to aid your healing process.

Rinse your eyes with eyebright and fennel tea, equal parts, for two to three weeks after surgery along with taking the following herbs internally.

Echinacea root—2 parts

Eyebright—2 parts

Goldenseal root—1 part

Calendula flowers—1 part

Comfrey root (optional)—1 part

Cleavers—1 part

Dose and Use: Take the tincture, 15–30 drops, two to three times per day with meals for ten to fourteen days following surgery.

I am most grateful for my friendship with Helen Nearing, author, and coauthor with Scott Nearing, of several books. Helen lives two hours north of me and I have many special memories of our times together. Helen has taught me a lot about love and kindness and living fully and dying well. The following quote is from her most recent book, *Loving and Leaving the Good Life.*

A network of love crisscrosses the globe. The delicate shining lines form a tenuous web from one end of the world to the other. There are so many threads of love in the world, so much love going on, for and from so many people. To have partaken of and to have given love is the greatest of life's rewards. There seems never an end to the loving that goes on forever and ever. Loving and leaving are a part of living.[6]

11

Immune-Enhancing Herbs

Every moment is enormous, and it is all we have.

—NATALIE GOLDBERG

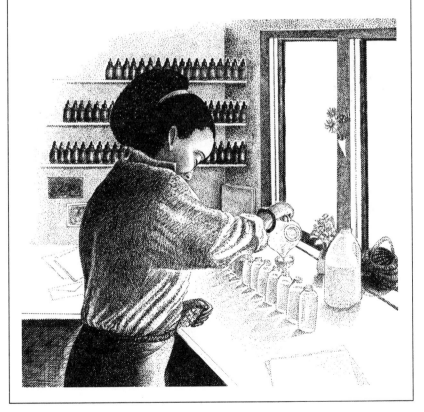

The immune system is intricately connected to all other systems in the body. Psychoneuroimmunology (PNI) is the term modern medicine has coined to describe the connection between mind and body; how the brain passes messages via the nerves to decrease or increase immune responses, and how emotions and thoughts affect these immune responses.

Keeping the immune system healthy means keeping the whole body (physical, emotional, mental, spiritual) healthy. For many people this includes unlearning the quick fix, popping-pill mentality that Western medicine sometimes teaches us. There are no shortcuts to acquiring health and happiness and no pills to miraculously "cure" a weakened immune system. The question to ask yourself when contemplating the health of your immune system is "How do I nourish myself?" Each person's body and life experiences are unique and what feeds and nourishes one person will vary for another. There are many different herbs to choose from and many health modalities to consider for increasing immune health.

Various herbs strengthen and rebuild the body's immune system. Some are effective for eliminating colds, swollen glands, and bacterial infections and work on a more surface level. Others work more deeply and stimulate the production of various immune cells through the bone marrow.[1] Still other herbs, such as liver tonics, support the liver and are important because Kupffer cells, found in the liver, destroy bacteria and other foreign substances that have been absorbed by the gastrointestinal tract. Some herbs help the various eliminative channels to function well, while other herbs offer us hope and uplift our spirits.

The ongoing process of relearning how to love oneself and to value being alive is an important part of restoring strength to our immune system and balance to Earth. Simple daily practices such as breathing deeply, praying, speaking kindly, treating ourselves and others compassionately, and making lifestyle changes that support a sustainable and nonviolent world, strengthen our spirits, our bodies, and our communities.

Nature offers us wisdom about how to live in harmony with ourselves and with the different seasons. When we resist and fight against the natural flow of nature, push ourselves as hard as we can, we become weak and more susceptible to dis-eases. An example of this can be seen by observing what plants and animals do during the wintertime in northern climates.

The season of winter is the time for inner reflection, for deeply resting and restoring our reserves for the coming seasons. Lots of plants become dormant in the winter, various animals hibernate. Many people are chronically exhausted because they do not allow themselves time to rest during the winter or are unable to because of socioeconomic factors. Replenishing our reserves each winter is essential for our overall health and vitality.

Dietary Support

Follow a simple, nourishing whole foods diet that includes dark leafy green vegetables, whole grains, sea vegetables, some legumes, and seasonal fruits. Eliminate white sugar and flour, fatty foods, alcohol, nicotine, and recreational drugs. Eat lots of garlic, drink at least four cups of nonchlorinated water a day along with various herb teas. Add 2–4 teaspoons of organic flax-seed oil, twice a day to vegetables, grains, or soup.

Supplements

Vitamin C–2000–3000 mg, two to three times a day. If you have an infection, work with an experienced health care provider at increasing your intake of vitamin C even more

Beta-carotene–75,000 IU, twice daily

Vitamin E–400 IU daily

Zinc–30 mg daily

A good quality B-complex vitamin

Blue-green algae tablets

Herbal Support

Echinacea purpurea and *Echinacea angustifolia* are the two most commonly used and commercially available echinacea species, though many more echinacea species grow in the United States, all of which are useful. Various Native American peoples informed white people about the uses of echinacea. Echinacea is effective in stimulating the immune response in various ways to ward off microbial infections and to increase the body's resistance to disease. Echinacea activates specific cells in the body to destroy cells overcome by viruses and other pathogens and also protects the plasma membranes of cells against viral attacks.

Over four hundred *Echinacea purpurea* plants grow in our medicinal herb gardens in Maine. They are beautiful perennials and winter well here in the north. The flowers bloom from mid-July to mid-September. They reseed themselves and are also easy to start from seed indoors in late March. The seed must be stratified (subjected to cold, moist conditions for one month) to break open the hard seed coat. I have found *Echinacea purpurea* to be much easier to start from seed than the *angustifolia* species. (Please note that because of its popularity, *Echinacea angustifolia* species are being overharvested in the wild. To ensure the survival of that species, ask for *Echinacea purpurea* or *Echinacea angustifolia* that is certified organically grown when buying dried root or tincture)

Echinacea plants grow slowly from seed and are often three to four inches high when we place them in the garden in late May. Native to the prairie, they prefer direct sun and well-drained soil. Echinacea leaves give a salad extra zing, as the fresh leaves have a tingly taste. My dog Mochi loves to take a few bites from the leaves. She doesn't consume them like cats do catnip, so you don't have to fear losing your echinacea plants to your dogs or cats.

To make echinacea flower tincture, we gather a few flowers from each plant and fill a glass jar, cover with grain alcohol and distilled water, and seal with a good-fitting lid. You can add fresh leaves to your tincture, but wait until your plants are three years old before digging the roots for tea or tincture. The seeds can also be chewed or tinctured.

Echinacea is a good remedy for the common cold, sore throats, swollen glands and lymph nodes, flu, infected cuts, mastitis, cystitis, vaginal infections, and infections of the upper respiratory tract and sinuses. I have found echinacea to be most effective in preventing a cold if taken before symptoms are full blown. When you feel a cold or infection coming on, take the tincture or tea every two hours until the acute symptoms lessen and then continue three to four times a day for seven to ten days. Take a break for a few days and continue for another ten days if needed.

If your body feels run down and vulnerable or if you are anticipating a stressful situation (traveling, exams, death of a loved one, moving) take echinacea three times a day for ten days, or take a smaller dose once a day, three to four times a week for several weeks or months. Echinacea is safe for pregnant and nursing women.

Many people ask if you can use echinacea over several months or years to keep the immune system strong. The latest research on echinacea suggests that it is most effective when used for specific situations and for ten-day intervals.[2] If you need to use it more than ten days, take a break for three days and repeat for another ten days. For chronic immune weakness, take smaller doses, 5–10 drops of tincture for adults, once a day for a few months along with other supportive herbs specific for your situation. Herbs used to stimulate the production of immune cells in the bone marrow are more effective for serious immune deficient illnesses than is echinacea and are discussed below.

Daily Immune Tonic

This formula is helpful for people who are not challenged with a specific immune deficient dis-ease, but wish to strengthen and maintain the health of their immune systems. The following herbs are appropriate for long-term use, slowly but surely rebuilding the energy deep within the body that many of us have depleted due to excessive or unhealthy lifestyles. Many of us also feel tired from living in these times when we are constantly assaulted with various kinds of pollution and the stresses of daily living.

Astragalus root—2 parts

Codonopsis root—2 parts
Siberian ginseng root—1 part
Schizandra berries—1 part
Prickly ash bark—1 part
Licorice root—½ part

Dose and Use: To make tea, soak 12 tablespoons of herbs overnight in 2 quarts of water and simmer, covered, for thirty to sixty minutes the following morning. Drink 1–3 cups per day. (Add in Siberian ginseng tincture if you cannot find good quality, dried Siberian ginseng roots, which in my experience are difficult to find on the commercial market) As a tincture, children can take 2–10 drops, one to two times per day, and adults can take 25–50 drops, one to two times per day. Take for at least two to six months to receive full benefit of these herbs and continue taking indefinitely as an immune tonic.

Note: These herbs should not be taken when acute symptoms flare up.

IMMUNE SUPPORT FOR COMPROMISED IMMUNE SYSTEMS

The following herbal formulas may be helpful for people who are HIV positive, have AIDS, cancer, chronic fatigue syndrome, or other conditions in which the immune system is severely compromised. These herbs improve the production of immune cells in the bone marrow; support the digestive system and improve assimilation of nutrients; help prevent frequent colds, flus, and other debilitating infections; and offer protection against the negative side effects of chemotherapy and radiation.

Long-Term Immune Support Herbs

Astragalus root—2 parts
Codonopsis root—1 part
Ligustrum berries—1 part

Siberian ginseng root—2 parts
Saw palmetto berries—1 part
Licorice root—1 part
Prickly ash bark—½ part

Dose and Use: To make tea, place 12 tablespoons of the herbs in 2 quarts of cool water and steep overnight. Simmer the mixture for thirty to forty minutes the following morning. Do not bother to strain off the herbs—let them continue to steep throughout the day. Drink 2–3 cups per day for many months. Add 10–20 drops of Siberian ginseng tincture to the tea unless you can find good quality Siberian ginseng roots. If taking the above herbs as a tincture, adults can take 25–50 drops, two to four times per day and children can take 5–10 drops, two to four times per day for several months.

Note: Do not take the above herbs during active stages of any infection, cold, or flu. Turn to specific herbs and other medications to help more quickly eliminate the infection and then resume the above herbs when the infection is gone.

Immune Response Stimulants

The following herbs stimulate the immune response and may be used for seven to ten days at a time when the immune system needs a stronger boost and for specific situations such as bronchitis, pneumonia, flus, candida, skin lesions, and colds. They may be considered along with other therapies for people with HIV, herpes, and chronic fatigue syndrome. Stay in good contact with your health care provider.

Lomatium—1 part
Usnea—1 part
Echinacea root—1 part

Goldenseal root—1 part

Dose and Use: As a tincture, take 25–50 drops, three to five times a day.

❀

Liver Herbs

The following herbs improve digestion and the assimilation of nutrients necessary for good health along with stimulating and strengthening the liver.

Dandelion root—
  2 parts
Blessed thistle—1
  part
Gentian root—1
  part
Burdock root—1 part
Wild yam root—1 part

Burdock

Dose and Use: As a tea, place 1 tablespoon of each of the roots into 1 quart of water and simmer twenty to thirty minutes, covered. Take off heat and add 1 tablespoon of blessed thistle and steep five to ten minutes, covered. Drink ¼–½ cup twenty minutes before meals. Or take the tincture, 20–40 drops, twenty minutes before meals.

Nervines

The following herbs help ease anxiety and stress, regulate nervous function, and uplift the spirit.

Oatstraw—2 parts
Skullcap—1 part
Borage leaves—1 part
Sacred basil—1 part
St. Johnswort—1 part
Lavender—1 part
Lemon balm—2 parts

Dose and Use: To make a tea, place 6 tablespoons in a glass quart jar, pour hot steaming water to the top of the jar, and seal with a good-fitting lid. Let steep ten to twenty minutes. Drink warm or cool throughout the day. For variety in flavor, occasionally mix with an unsweetened fruit juice and squirt of lemon juice.

Stay in good contact with an experienced herbalist and other health care providers. You may need to change the formulas from time to time to support the changes in your body. Look for a well-trained Chinese herbalist or acupuncturist in your area. People trained in traditional Chinese medicine have a good understanding of the overall body and not just symptoms. They can diagnose which organs are weakened and are skilled in how to strengthen them and how to rebuild the whole body instead of focusing on wiping out the "disease."

For people with HIV or AIDS, I recommend listening to an excellent talk by herbalist Amanda McQuade Crawford called "Wholeness, Herbs, and AIDS" available by mail by writing Amanda at P.O. Box 66, Ojai, California, 93024. Look for her upcoming book on herbal therapies for AIDS called *By a Revolution of Consciousness.*

HERBS AND VACCINATIONS

Research continues to show that vaccinations attack and weaken the immune system. If you choose to be vaccinated take tinctures or teas of echinacea root, astragalus root, and northern white cedar (*Thuja occidentalis*) twigs or chew on fresh cedar twigs. All of these strengthen the body and help counteract side effects of vaccinations. Take the tincture or tea three to four times per day, seven days before, the day of, and seven days after being immunized along with daily doses of vitamin C. Homeopathic doctors also have various remedies they recommend to help counteract side effects of vaccinations.

Cedar

Note: Pregnant women should avoid cedar because of its strong emmenagogue properties.

Researchers are investigating various homeopathic remedies, called nosodes, as alternatives to various vaccinations. You may want to further investigate this with a homeopathic vet or in homeopathic journals before you, your children, or your animals are vaccinated. I am using nosodes with my dog and cat instead of vaccinations.

Fever/Flu Remedy

The following formula is one of my favorites for quickly vitalizing the immune system to ward off colds, flus, and other viral infections of the respiratory tract. They also relieve achy feelings that often accompany a cold or flu, and help reduce fevers.

Boneset flowers and leaves—2 parts
White yarrow flowers—2 parts
Horehound flowers and leaves—1 part
Calendula flowers—1 part
Mullein leaves—2 parts

Dose and Use: Use as a tea or tincture. The tea is bitter tasting and can be difficult for children and some adults to take. For acute symptoms, children can take 2–5 drops of tincture or ⅛–½ cup tea every one to two hours; adults 25–50 drops of tincture or 1 cup of tea every one to two hours until acute phase diminishes. Continue using the same amount of drops, three times a day for at least seven to ten days after the acute symptoms have subsided, or longer if needed.

ENVIRONMENTAL ILLNESSES

There are a growing number of health problems being linked to various pesticides and toxic substances, including exposure to chemical warfare, radioactive waste, and other industrial pollutants. As I am finishing this book various news reports are coming out about strange cancers and other diseases veterans from the Desert Storm war are being diagnosed with. The Pentagon says there is not enough evidence to prove these women and men were exposed to biological and/or chemical warfare and therefore their medical bills are not being paid for by the United States government.

Terry Tempest Williams writes in *Refuge: An Unnatural History of Family and Place*, about her mother's journey with breast cancer due to exposure to nuclear testing near Salt Lake City, Utah, and her own journey with wondering if she herself will be diagnosed with breast cancer someday—a question that haunts thousands of women today.

Jim Hightower, former agricultural commissioner of Texas, writes in a small article titled "Breast Cancer's Chemical Connection":

Evidence is growing that a line of manmade chemicals called organochlorines is the chief villain in the rise of this cancer, which now kills fifty thousand American women each year. Used to make everything from pesticides to plastics, hundreds of organochlorines are now known to cause cancer. And the higher your exposure to these toxins, the higher your chances are of getting cancer. One tidbit: Look to Israel. Prior to 1976, this small nation was soaked in organochlorine pesticides, and Israeli women suffered about the highest rate of breast cancer deaths in the world. So, in '78, their government launched an aggressive program banning those pesticides. The result? Israel's rate of deaths due to this killer sharply decreased—while the death rate in every other nation continued to increase. But in our country, guess who are major funders and players inside most cancer research institutions? None other than the corporations that make and use organochlorines. So our medical establishment busies itself with trying to cure breast cancer, rather than preventing it.[4]

Rachel Carson, author of *Silent Spring*, published in 1962, helped expose the dangerous health hazards of DDT and other pesticides. Have the manufacturers of pesticides, huge chemical farmers, the United States government, and consumers listened to her warnings? Songbirds and other migratory birds continue to die because of exposure to heavy metals and other toxins and from being sucked down huge smokestacks of factories. It is spring as I complete the writing of this book. I have a heavy heart as I do not hear many songs outside my window. Every year I think perhaps they are just slow to return. So I turn my attention to the return of the hummingbirds. I hope they will always return, just as I hope there will always be dandelions to dig in spring.

There are various herbs and foods that can be used to detoxify the body from various environmental toxins. Through Avena Botanicals, I have produced a number of herbal tinctures formulated by a very fine herbalist, Hart Brent, from Peacham, Vermont, who works with many people exposed to toxins. These formulas are effective, yet are not the cure to environmental illnesses.

When I think of helping lessen environmental pollution I think about improving the health of the soil that grows food and herbs because I have always been connected to land. I am fortunate to still be land based, living next to a six-thousand-acre protected wetland. I do not know how to solve the massive social and environmental problems we face. But I do believe one area to focus in on is helping large and small farmers and backyard gardeners relearn how to care for the soil by appropriate and sustainable farming practices. When pesticide-free food grown in our bioregions is the standard food available at affordable prices, we will see the health of humans, animals, and plant species; the water, air, and Earth herself become healthier. As we begin to heal the wounds that have left us disconnected from Earth and isolated from ourselves and other living species, we can help our communities make changes to assure an unpolluted and green future.

Afterword

Many people waited patiently, some even anxiously, for this book. In the four and a half years it took me to complete it, many changes occurred within me. The writing process itself was a profound inner journey. The book is a better book today because of its long gestation.

I wish to honor three women, mentioned in this book, who passed on into the spirit world during the writing of this book. My dear friend and teacher since I was nineteen years old, Adele Dawson; Marija Gimbutas, whose belief in me and in the healing potential of herbs was invaluable; and Nancy Devine, whose two poems grace this book. Nancy took her own life once the ice left a pond near her home as this book came to completion—a powerful reminder of the enormous pain and isolation many women feel. It is my hope that the world of herbs will once again reconnect all of us with Earth, reminding us that we are deeply loved by her.

Resources

Artemis Speaks: V. B. A. C. Stories and Natural Childbirth Information, by Nan Koehler. Occidental, CA: Jerald R. Brown, 1985. (Available from Jerald R. Brown, Inc., 17440 Taylor Lane, Occidental, CA 95465.)

Gaiacology, by Amanda McQuade Crawford. Freedom, CA: Crossing Press, forthcoming, 1995.

Gynecology and Naturopathic Medicine: A Treatment Manual, by Tori Hudson, N.D. Beaverton, OR: TK Publications, 1992. (Available for health care providers from TK Publications, 19153 Butternut Drive, Beaverton, OR 97007.)

Healing Yourself During Pregnancy, by Joy Gardner. Freedom, CA: Crossing Press, 1990.

Herbal Healing for Women, by Rosemary Gladstar. New York, NY: Simon & Schuster, 1993.

Natural Healing in Gynecology, by Rina Nissim. New York, NY: Pandora Press, 1986.

Natural Medicine for Women, by Julian and Susan Scott. New York, NY: Avon Books, 1991.

Vitex: The Women's Herb, by Christopher Hobbs. Capitola, CA: Botanica Press, 1990.

The Wise Woman Herbal for the Childbearing Years, by Susun Weed. Woodstock, NY: Ash Tree Publishing, 1986.

The Wise Woman Herbal for the Menopausal Years, by Susun Weed. Woodstock, NY: Ash Tree Publishing, 1992.

Witches Heal: Lesbian Herbal Self-Sufficiency, by Billie Potts. Bearsville, NY: Hecuba's Daughters, Inc., 1981.

GENERAL WOMEN'S HEALTH BOOKS

A New View of a Woman's Body, by the Federation of Feminist Women's Health Centers. New York, NY: Simon & Schuster, 1981.

The Black Women's Health Book: Speaking for Ourselves, edited by Evelyn C. White. Seattle, WA: Seal Press, 1990.

Dr. Susan Love's Breast Book, by Susan M. Love, M.D., with Karen Lindsey. Reading, MA: Addison-Wesley, 1991.

Changing Bodies, Changing Lives, by Ruth Bell, and other coauthors of *Our Bodies, Ourselves* and *Ourselves and Our Children*, and with members of the Teen Book Project. New York, NY: Vintage Books, 1988.

A Difficult Decision: A Compassionate Book About Abortion, by Joy Gardner, which offers compassionate insights and alternative information for women looking for support in terminating a pregnancy. Crossing Press, P.O. Box 1048, Freedom, CA 95019.

Fibroid Tumors and Endometriosis: A Self-Help Program, by Susan M. Lark, M.D. Los Altos, CA: Westchester Publishing Company, 1993.

The New Our Bodies, Ourselves, by the Boston Women's Health Book Collective. New York, NY: Simon & Schuster, 1992.

Ourselves, Growing Older, by Paula Brown Doress and Diana Laskin Siegal. New York, NY: Simon & Schuster, 1987.

Premenstrual Syndrome Self-Help Book, by Susan Lark, M.D. Los Angeles, CA: Forman Publishing, 1984.

Self-Ritual for Invoking Release of Spirit Life in the Womb by Deborah Maia. This book offers alternative insights for women looking for support in terminating a pregnancy. Mother Spirit Publishing, P.O. Box 893, Great Barrington, MA 01230.

Women of the Fourteenth Moon: Women Writing on Menopause, edited by Dena Taylor and Amber Coverdale Sumrall. Capitola, CA: Crossing Press, 1991.

Woman: Your Body, Your Health: The Essential Guide for Well-Being, by Josleen Wilson. San Diego, CA: Harcourt Brace Jovanovich, 1990.

Women's Health: Readings on Social, Economic, and Political Issues, by Nancy Worcester and Marianne H. Whately. Dubuque, IA: Kendall/Hunt Publishing Co., 1988.

Women's Bodies, Women's Wisdom, by Christine Northrup, M.D. New York, NY: Bantam, 1994.

LESBIAN HEALTH BOOKS AND RESOURCES

Alive and Well, A Lesbian Health Guide, by Cuca Hepburn and B. Gutierrez. Freedom, CA: Crossing Press, 1988.

Dykes, Disability, and Stuff, a national quarterly newsletter. (Available from Catherine Lohr, P.O. Box 6194, Boston, MA 02114.)

Homophobia: A Weapon of Sexism, by Susanne Pharr. Inverness, CA: Chardon Press, 1988.

Lambda Resource Center for the Blind, recordings of books for lesbians and gay men. (3225 N. Sheffield Ave., Chicago, IL 60657 (312) 274–0510.)

Lesbian Health Matters!, by Mary O'Donnell, et al. (Published in 1979 by, and available from, Santa Cruz Women's Health Center, 250 Locust St., Santa Cruz, CA 95060.)

Lesbian Passion: Loving Ourselves and Each Other, by JoAnn Loulan. San Francisco, CA: Spinsters/Aunt Lute Book Co., 1987.

National Lesbian Health Care Survey, 1988, a report of the findings of a national study of lesbian health care needs and concerns. (National Lesbian and Gay Health Foundation, P.O. Box 65472, Washington, DC 20035.)

MEDICINAL HERB BOOKS

American Materia Medica: Therapeutics and Pharmacognosy, edited by Finely Ellingwood. Portland, OR: Eclectic Medical Publications,

1983. (Available from Eclectic Medical Publications, 11231 S.E. Market St., Portland, OR 97212.)

Between Heaven and Earth, by Efrem Korngold and Harriet Beinfield. New York, NY: Ballantine Books, 1991.

The Complete Book of Essential Oils and Aromatherapy, by Valerie Ann Worwood. San Rafael, CA: New World Library, 1991.

The Complete Medicinal Herbal, by Penelope Ody. New York, NY: Dorling Kindersley, 1993.

Discovering Wild Plants, by Janice Schofield. Anchorage, AK: Northwest Books, 1989.

Earthmagic: Finding and Using Medicinal Herbs, by Corrine Martin. Woodstock, VT: Country Man Press, 1991.

An Elder's Herbal: Natural Techniques for Promoting Health and Vitality, by David Hoffman. Rochester, VT: Healing Arts Press, 1993.

The Encyclopedia of Herbs and Herbalism, edited by Malcolm Stuart. London: MacDonald and Co., 1987.

The Family Herbal, by Barbara and Peter Theiss. Rochester, VT: Healing Arts Press, 1989.

Flower Esssence Repertory, by Patricia Kaminski and Richard Katz. Nevada City, CA: Flower Essence Society, updated 1992.

Foundations of Health: The Liver and Digestive Herbal, by Christopher Hobbs. Capitola, CA: Botanica Press, 1992.

Guide to Medicinal Plants, by Paul Schauenberg and Ferdinand Paris. New Canaan, CT: Keats Publishing, 1977.

Herbal Body Book, by Jeanne Rose. New York, NY: Putnam Publishing Group, 1976.

Herbal Medicine, by Rudolf Fritz Weiss, M.D. Beaconsfield, England: Beaconsfield Publishers, 1988. (U.S. distributor: Medicina Biologica, Portland, OR 97212.)

Herbs, by Roger Phillips and Nicky Foy. London, England: Pan Books, 1990.

Herbs for Common Ailments, by Anne McIntyre. New York, NY: Simon & Schuster, 1992.

The Herbs of Life, by Lesley Tierra. Freedom, CA: Crossing Press, 1992.

Herbs: Partners in Life, by Adele Dawson. Rochester, VT: Healing Arts Press, 1991.

The Holistic Herbal, by David Hoffman. Scotland: Findhorn Press, 1983.

The Illustrated Herbal Encyclopedia, by Kathi Keville. New York, NY: Bantam Doubleday, 1992.

King's American Dispensatory, edited by Harvey W. Felter. Portland, OR: Eclectic Medical Publications, 1983. (Available from Eclectic Medical Publications, 11231 S.E. Market St. Portland, OR 97212.)

Medicinal and Other Uses of North American Plants: A Historical Survey with Special Reference to the Eastern Indian Tribes, by Charlotte Erichsen-Brown. New York, NY: Dover Publications, 1979.

Medicinal Plants of the Desert and Canyon West, by Michael Moore. Santa Fe, NM: Museum of New Mexico Press, 1989.

Medicinal Plants of the Mountain Southwest, by Michael Moore. Santa Fe, NM: Museum of New Mexico Press, 1979.

Medicines From the Earth: A Guide to Healing Plants, edited by William Thompson, M.D. Maidenhead, England: McGraw-Hill Book Company (UK), 1978.

Micmac Medicines: Remedies and Recollections, by Laurie Lacey. Halifax, Nova Scotia: Nimbus Publishing Co, 1993.

A Modern Herbal, by Maude Grieve., 2 volumes, New York, NY: Dover Publications, 1971.

Native Harvests: Recipes and Botanicals of the American Indian, by Barrie Kavasch. New York, NY: Random House, 1979.

The New Age Herbalist, by Richard Mabey. New York, NY: Collier Books/Macmillan, 1988.

Planetary Herbology: An Integration of Western Herbs into the Traditional Chinese and Ayurvedic Systems, by Michael Tierra. Santa Fe, NM: Lotus Press, 1988.

Roots: An Underground Botany and Forager's Guide, by Douglas B. Elliott. Old Greenwich, CT: Chatman Press, 1976.

Tree Medicine Tree Magic, by Ellen Evert Hopman. Custer, WA: Phoenix Publishing, 1991.

Usnea: The Herbal Antibiotic, by Christopher Hobbs. Capitola, CA: Botanica Press, 1986.

WOMEN'S SPIRITUALITY AND EARTH-CENTERED BOOKS

Anoqcou: Ceremony Is Life Itself, by gkisedtanamoogk and Frances Hancock. Portland, ME: Astarte Shell Press, 1993.

The Attentive Heart: Conversations with Trees, by Stephanie Kaza. New York, NY: Ballantine Books, 1993.

The Civilization of the Goddess: The World of Old Europe, by Marija Gimbutas. San Francisco, CA: HarperCollins, 1991.

Dreaming the Dark: Magic, Sex and Politics, by Starhawk. Boston, MA: Beacon Press, 1982.

For Her Own Good: 150 Years of the Experts' Advice to Women, by Barbara Ehrenreich and Deirdre English. New York, NY: Doubleday, 1978.

Glory! To the Flowers, by Maggie Steincrohn Davis. Blue Hill, ME: Heartsong Books, forthcoming, March 1995.

Healing the Wounds: The Promise of Ecofeminism, edited by Judith Plant. Philadelphia, PA: New Society Publishers, 1989.

The Language of the Goddess, by Marija Gimbutas. London, England: Thames and Hudson, 1989.

Learning True Love: How I Learned and Practiced Social Change in Vietnam, by Cao Ngoc Phuong. Berkeley, CA: Parallax Press, 1993.

Long Quiet Highway: Waking Up In America, by Natalie Goldberg. New York, NY: Bantam Books, 1992.

Love In Action: Writings on Nonviolent Social Change, by Thich Nhat Hanh. Berkeley, CA: Parallax Press, 1993.

Loving and Leaving the Good Life, by Helen Nearing. Post Mills, VT: Chelsea Green Publishing Company, 1992.

Medicine Women, Curanderas, and Women Doctors, by Bobette Perrone, H. Henrietta Stockel, and Victoria Krueger. Norman, OK and London, England: University of Oklahoma Press, 1989.

Shakti Woman: Feeling Our Fire, Healing Our World, the New Female

Shamanism, by Vicki Noble. New York, NY: HarperCollins, 1991.

Sister Outsider: Essays and Speeches, by Audre Lorde. Trumansburg, NY: Crossing Press, 1984.

States of Grace: The Recovery of Meaning in the Postmodern Age, by Charlene Spretnak. New York, NY: Harper San Francisco, 1991.

Touching Peace: Practicing the Art of Mindful Living, by Thich Nhat Hanh. Berkeley, CA: Parallax Press, 1992.

Through the Goddess: A Woman's Way of Healing, by Patricia Reis. New York, NY: Continuum, 1991.

When God Was a Woman, by Merlin Stone. San Diego, CA: Harcourt Brace Jovanovich, 1976.

Witches, Midwives, and Nurses, by Barbara Ehrenreich and Deirdre English. Old Westbury, NY: Feminist Press, 1973.

Woman and Nature: The Roaring Inside Her, by Susan Griffin. New York, NY: Harper & Row, 1978.

Woman as Healer: A Panoramic Survey of the Healing Activities of Women From Prehistoric Times to the Present, by Jeanne Achterberg. Boston, MA: Shambala Publications, 1990.

BOOKS ON HOMEOPATHY

The Complete Homeopathy Handbook, by Miranda Castro. New York, NY: St. Martin's Press, 1990. (This is a favorite of mine.)

Everybody's Guide to Homeopathic Medicine, by Stephen Cummings and Dana Ullman. Los Angeles, CA: Jeremy P. Tarcher, Inc., 1991.

Homeopathic Medicines for Pregnancy and Childbirth, by Richard Moskowitz, M.D. Berkeley, CA: North Atlantic Books and Homeopathic Educational Services, 1992.

Homeopathy for Pregnancy, Birth, and Your Baby's First Year, by Miranda Castor. New York, NY: St. Martin's Press, 1992.

Pocket Manual of Homeopathic Materia Medica with Repertory and Indian Drugs, by William Boericke, M.D. New Delhi, India: B. Jain Publishers, 1991.

Portraits of Homeopathic Medicines: Psychophysical Analyses of Selected Constitutional Types, by Catherine Coulter. Berkeley, CA: North Atlantic Books, volume 1, 1986; volume 2, 1988.

The Science of Homeopathy, by George Vithoulkas. New York, NY: Grove Press, 1980.

SUPPLIERS OF BOOKS AND TAPES ON HOMEOPATHY

Homeopathic Educational Services
2124 Kettredege St.
Berkeley, CA 94704
(800) 359–9051 (9–6, Pacific time)
Books and tapes

The Minimum Price
795 Peace Portola Dr., Suite AA
Blaine, WA 98230
(800) 663–8272

GENERAL HEALTH BOOKS

Encyclopedia of Natural Medicine, by Michael Murray, N.D., and Joseph Pizzorno, N.D. Rocklin, CA: Prima Publishing, 1991.

Fighting Radiation With Foods, Herbs, and Vitamins, by Steven Schechter, N.D. Brookline, MA: East West Health Books, 1988.

Staying Healthy With Nutrition, by Elson M. Haas, M.D., Berkeley, CA: Celestial Arts, 1992.

Staying Healthy With the Seasons, by Elson M. Haas, M.D., Berkeley, CA: Celestial Arts, 1981.

COOKBOOKS

May All Be Fed: Diet For a New World, by John Robbins. New York, NY: Avon Books, 1992.

The Peaceful Cook, by Harriet Kofalk. Summertown, TN: The Book Publishing Co., 1991.

The Self-Healing Cookbook, by Kristina Turner. Grass Valley, CA: Earthtones Press, 1987.

GARDENING BOOKS

Botany for Gardeners: An Introduction and Guide, by Brian Capon. Portland, OR: Timber Press, 1990.

The Complete Book of Everlastings: Growing, Drying, and Designing With Dried Flowers, by Mark and Terry Silber. New York, NY: Alfred A. Knopf, 1988.

Culture and Horticulture: A Philosophy of Gardening, by Wolf D. Storl. Wyoming, RI: Bio-Dynamic Literature, 1979.

Dictionary of Plant Names, by Allen Coombes. Portland, OR: Timber Press, 1985.

The Garden Primer, by Barbara Damrosch. New York, NY: Workman Publishing Group, 1988.

Garden Variety Dykes: Lesbian Traditions in Gardening, an Anthology, edited by Irene Reti and Valerie Jean Chase. Santa Cruz, CA: Her Books, 1994.

Hedgemaids and Fairy Candles: The Lives and Lore of North American Wildflowers, by Jack Sanders. Camden, ME: Ragged Mountain Press, 1993.

Herbal Renaissance: Growing, Using and Understanding Herbs in the Modern World, by Steven Foster. Salt Lake City, UT: Gibbs Smith, Publisher, 1993.

Making a White Garden, by Joan Clifton. New York, NY, Grove Press, 1990.

Mandala Gardens, by Tarthang Tulku. Oakland, CA: Dharma Publishing, 1991.

The New Organic Grower's Four Season Harvest, by Eliot Coleman. Post Mills, VT: Chelsea Green Publishing, 1992.

Seeds of Change: The Living Treasure; The Passionate Story of the Growing Movement to Restore Biodiversity and Revolutionize the Way We Think About Food, by Kenny Ausubel. San Francisco, CA: HarperCollins, 1994.

Start With the Soil: The Organic Gardener's Guide to Improving Soil for Higher Yields, More Beautiful Flowers, and a Healthy, Easy-Care Garden, by Grace Gershuny. Emmaus, PA: Rodale Press, 1993.

Sunflower Houses: Garden Discoveries for Children of All Ages, by Sharon Lovejoy. Loveland, CO: Interweave Press, 1991.

Theme Gardens: How to Plan, Plant and Grow Sixteen Gloriously Different Gardens, by Barbara Damrosch. New York, NY: Workman Publishing, 1982.

Women's Health Resources

American Anorexia Nervosa Association, Inc.
418 E. 76th Street
New York, NY 10021
(212) 734-1114

or

Anorexia Nervosa and Related Eating Disorders, Inc.
P.O. Box 5102
Eugene, OR 97405
(503) 344-1144
Either of the two above groups can direct you to a support group near you.

Boston Women's Health Information Center
240A Elm Street
Somerville, MA 02144
(617) 625-0271
In addition to its well-known sourcebook, *Our Bodies, Ourselves,* the collective also makes available packets of information on menopause, osteoporosis, cardiovascular disease, and hormone replacement therapy. This is the organization to contact for health information and resources on a variety of women's health issues and multicultural women's health concerns.

National Alliance of Breast Cancer Organizations (NABCO)
1180 Avenue of the Americas, 2nd floor
New York, NY 10036
(212) 221-3300
Contact for Breast Cancer Coalition; provides written information, resources.

MEDITATION RESOURCES

Community of Mindful Living
P.O. Box 7355
Berkeley, CA 94704
Publishes *The Mindfulness Bell*, a newsletter by friends and students of Vietnamese Buddhist teacher Thich Nhat Hanh. Thich Nhat Hanh's yearly retreat and teaching schedule is listed in *The Mindfulness Bell*.

HIV/AIDS RESOURCES AND ORGANIZATIONS

AIDS: Alternative Approaches to the Understanding and the Treatment of Aquired Immune Deficiency Syndrome Based on Anthroposophilical Medicine, by Arie Bos. Stroud, United Kingdom: Hawthorn Press, 1989.

AIDS: Passageway to Transformation, by C. Norman Shealy, M.D., Ph.D., and Caroline M. Myss. Walpole, NH: Stillpoint Publishing, 1987.

Women, AIDS and Activism, by the ACT UP/New York Women and AIDS Book Group. Boston, MA: South End Press, 1990.

The Positive Woman: A Newsletter By, For, and About the HIV Positive Woman.
P.O. Box 34372
Washington, DC 20043-4372
(202) 898-0372

ACT UP (AIDS Coalition to Unleash Power)
135 West 29th Street, Suite 10
New York, NY 10001
(212) 564-2437
AIDS activist organization.

National AIDS Hot Line
(800) 342-AIDS
Spanish: (800) 344-7432
TTY: (800) 243-7889
National and local referral. TTY line is open Monday through

Friday, 10:00 A.M. to 10:00 P.M., EST. Spanish line available from 8:00 A.M. to 2:00 A.M., seven days a week. English line is open twenty-four hours a day, 365 days a year.

HERBAL EDUCATIONAL RESOURCES

Amanda McQuade Crawford, former Findhorn gardener and herbal practitioner with a diploma in phytotherapy from Britain's National Institute of Medical Herbalists offers a variety of herb courses. Write her at P.O. Box 66, Ojai, CA 93024.

American Herb Association (AHA)
P.O. Box 1673
Nevada City, CA 95959
   Publishes a wonderful and informative newsletter and directories of herb classes and correspondence courses in the United States.

American Herbalist Guild (AHG)
P.O. Box 1127
Forestville, CA 95436
   Publishes a newsletter for members and a directory of herb classes and practitioners.

Avena Institute
20 Mill Street
Rockland, ME 04841
(207) 594–0694
   Founded by me, Deb Soule, in 1990. Avena Institute is a nonprofit, multicultural education center. Our teaching focuses on skills that help people live respectfully with Earth and all life forms. Specific programs include a monthly herb class for six months for women, wild herb walks, organic gardening, special herb walks led by me in my beautiful one-acre medicinal herb gardens, herbal animal care, and crosscultural exchanges. We print a yearly teaching schedule every winter.

Blazing Star Herbal School
P.O. Box 6
Shelburne Falls, MA 01370
   Gail Ulrich, wise woman herbalist and flower essence practi-

tioner, offers a variety of herbal classes and organizes the annual East Coast Women's Herb Conference.

Green Terrestrial
P.O. Box 41
Milton, NY 12547

Pam Montgomery, spirited and wise woman herbalist, offers a variety of herbal classes and organizes the annual Green Nations Gathering.

New Mexico Herb Center
122 Tulane SE
Albuquerque, NM 87106
(505) 265-2631

Offers a nine-month medicinal herb course with clinical training.

Northeast Herbal Association
P.O. Box 146
Marshfield, VT 05658-0146

A wonderful organization that publishes a newsletter and booklet that lists herbalists and herbal activities in the eastern United States.

The Science and Art of Herbalism: A Home Study Course by
Rosemary Gladstar
P.O. Box 420
East Barre, VT 05649

A beautifully written mail-order course for students who wish to gain a deeper and systematic understanding of herbs that includes wildcrafting, herbal preparation, formulation, earth awareness, and respect for the spirit of the plants. Rosemary also offers a variety of herb classes and seminars at her home in Vermont.

The School of Herbal Medicine (American branch of the School of Herbal Medicine-Phytotherapy, England) offers a correspondence course. Send business-size SASE to P.O. Box 168-C, Squamish, WA 98392.

Therapeutic Herbalism, by David Hoffman

An in-depth correspondence course focused on the clinical application of medicinal herbs. David's well-organized class material is available with or without the course and well worth the price.

For more information write David Hoffman, 9304 Spring Hill School Rd., Sebastapol, CA 95472.

Wild Rose College of Natural Healing offers a full-time, three-year clinical training for herbalists. Send $5 money order with return address to WWRC, 1745 West 4th Ave., Vancouver, BC V6J1M2, Canada, or call (604) 734–4596.

Wise Woman herbal medicine classes and workshops offered by Susun Weed, P.O. Box 64, Woodstock, NY 12498.

HERBAL NEWSLETTERS

The American Herb Association Newsletter
P.O. Box 1673
Nevada City, CA 95959

Foster's Botanical and Herb Reviews
P.O. Box 106
Eureka Springs, AR 72632

HerbalGram
P.O. Box 201660
Austin, TX 78720

Herb Companion
201 East Fourth St.
Loveland, CO 80537

The Herb Quarterly
P.O. Box 548
Boiling Springs, PA 17007

Medical Herbalism
P.O. Box 33080
Portland, OR 97233

NEHA
The Northeast Herb Association
P.O. Box 146
Marshfield, VT 05658

Protocol Journal of Botanical Medicines
A peer-reviewed publication offering current and thoroughly refer-enced material for use in both clinical and educational settings. Call (800) 852–6271.

MEDICINAL HERB SOURCES

The following small businesses offer very good quality herbs and herbal products.

Avena Botanicals
20 Mill St.
Rockland, ME 04841

I started Avena Botanicals in 1985 because of the need for organically grown and wild-harvested medicinal herb products in Maine. We make special remedies for women and animals: teas, oils, salves, and over 150 tinctures and offer them through our mail-order catalog and through various food co-ops, health food stores, and health care providers. The majority of the herbs we use are carefully grown and gathered in Avena's one-acre gardens and from nearby fields, woods, and islands.

Green Terrestrial
P.O. Box 41
Milton, NY 12547

Herbalist Pam Montgomery makes a line of herbal products from organic and wild herbs and offers them through her mail-order catalog.

Herbalist and Alchemist
P.O. Box 458
Bloomsbury, NJ 12547

Herbalist David Winston offers good-quality herbal products and a variety of high-quality dried Chinese herbs through his mail-order catalog.

The Herb Closet
104 Main St.
Montpelier, VT 05602

A wonderful shop to visit or order from. A collectively owned and operated business with a large selection of tinctures, dried herbs, capsules, and books.

Island Herbs
Waldron Island, WA 98297

Herbalist and botanist Ryan Drum wildcrafts herbs and collects a variety of sea vegetables that are of excellent quality. Write him for his current price list and availability.

Maine Coast Sea Vegetables
Franklin, ME 04634
   Sells exceptionally high-quality sea vegetables in bulk and a variety of delicious sea vegetable products. Retail and wholesale.

Pacific Botanicals
4350 Fish Hatchery Rd.
Grants Pass, OR 97527
   Excellent selection of certified organic fresh and dried herbs by the pound, catalog available.

Sage Mountain Herb Products
P.O. Box 420
East Barre, VT 05649
   A small, family-run business that offers high-quality herbal tinctures and products formulated by herbalist Rosemary Gladstar, who is a gifted and experienced herbalist.

Wise Woman Herbals
P.O. Box 328
Gladstone, OR 97027
   Naturopathic doctor Sharol Tilgner offers a line of herbal extracts, vaginal suppositories, capsules, and solid extracts.

FLOWER ESSENCES

Flower Essence Services
P.O. Box 459
Nevada City, CA 95959
   They offer several hundred types of flower essences along with wonderful books and pure essential oils.

Flowers of the Soul
Hart Brent
P.O. Box 75
W. Danville, VT 05873
(802) 684–2570
   Hart is a gifted herbal practitioner and creator of the Flowers of

the Soul, which captures the essence of compassion and helps one move through their soul's journey with self-love and universal love.

Green Hope Farm
P.O. Box 125
Meriden, NH 03770
    Special essences made by Molly Sheehan from flowers from Bermuda, the Adirondack mountains, and her own magical gardens.

Running Fox Farm
74 Thrasher Hill Rd
Worthington, MA 01098
    Flower essences made by a lovely woman, Katherin Landry.

Woodland Flower Essences
Kate and Don Gilday
P.O. Box 125
Wendell, MA 01379
    As of spring 1995 write them at Cold Brook, NY 13324. Joyful and spirited herbalist Kate and her partner, Don, a gifted woodworker, have created a special set of flower essences made from tree, shrub, and the forest floor flowers.

PLANT AND SEED RESOURCES

Abundant Life Seed Foundation
P.O. Box 772
Port Townsend, WA 98368
    Retail catalog $1 and bulk price list, good source of organic heirlooms, good book section.

Bountiful Gardens
18001 Shafer Ranch Rd.
Willits, CA 95490
    Educational projects and organic seeds.

Companion Plants
7297 North Coolville Ridge Rd.
Athens, OH 45701
    Huge selection of medicinal herb plants.

The Cook's Garden
P.O. Box 65
Londonderry, VT 05418
Catalog $1, specializing in salad greens and varieties for new cuisine.

Elixir Farm Botanicals
Brixey, MO 65618
Chinese and indigenous medicinal plant seeds.

Fedco Seeds
P.O. Box 520
Waterville, ME 04903
Cooperative offering seeds, tubers, and trees for cold climates.

The Flower and Herb Exchange
3076 N. Winn Rd.
Decorah, IA 52101
One thousand varieties of heirloom herbs and flowers, annual membership $5.

Forest Farm
990 Tetherow Rd.
Williams, OR 97544
Write them for their catalog of their large selection of trees.

Garden City Seeds
1324 Red Crow Rd.
Victor, MT 598875
Retail catalog $2 and bulk price list, oriented to cold climates, very economical.

Halcyon Gardens Herbs
P.O. Box 75
Wexford, PA 15090
Catalog $2, herbs and herb garden kits.

High Altitude Gardens
P.O. Box 1048
Hailey, ID 83333
Catalog $3, oriented to high altitudes and cold climates.

Hsu's Ginseng Enterprises, Inc.
T6819 County Highway
W. Wausau, WI 54401
   Seeds and rootlets.

J.L. Hudson, Seedsman
P.O. Box 1058
Redwood City, CA 94064
   Catalog $1, best selection of unusual cultivars.

Johnny's Selected Seeds
310 Foss Hill Rd.
Albion, ME 04910
   Excellent research and cultural information.

J.W. Jung Seed Co.
335 S. High St.
Randolph, WI 53957
Interesting cultivars.

The Landis Valley Museum
2451 Kissel Hill Rd.
Lancaster, PA 17601
   Catalog $2, heirlooms grown by Amish and Mennonites before
World War II.

Maine Organic Farmers and Gardeners Association (MOFGA)
P.O. Box 2176
Augusta, ME 04338
   Works to promote sustainable agriculture through educational
and legislative initiatives, write for membership information.

Native Seeds/SEARCH
2509 N. Campbell #325
Tucson, AZ 85719
   Catalog $1, traditional Native American crops.

Nature's Cathedral
R.R. #1, Box 120
Blairstown, IA 52209
   Supplier of excellent quality organic and wild-harvested medic-
inal herbs.

Nichols Garden Nursery
1190 North Pacific Hwy.
Albany, OR 97321
    Herbs and novelty varieties.

Northeast Organic Farming Association (NOFA)
Julie Rawson
RFD 2 Sheldon Rd.
Barre, MA 01005
    Write for information about membership and educational activities on sustainable agriculture in Massachusetts, Connecticut, New York, Vermont, New Hampshire, Rhode Island, and New Jersey.

Otto Richter & Sons
Goodwood Ontario, Canada LOC 1AO
    Huge selection of interesting medicinal herb seeds.

Peace Seeds
P.O. Box 190
Gila, NM 88038
    Catalog $4, organic and wildcrafted seed for unusual cultivars.

Pinetree Garden Seeds
Route 100
New Gloucester, ME 04260
    Small packets for the home gardener.

Sandy Mush Herb Nursery
316 Surrett Cove Rd.
Leicester, NC 28748-9622
    1100 varieties of herbs, flowering perennials, dye plants, and unusual trees and shrubs.

Seeds Blum
Idaho City Stage
Boise, ID 83706
    Catalog $3, heirlooms.

Seeds of Change
1364 Rufina Circle #5
Santa Fe, NM 87501
    Catalog $3, organic seeds.

Seed Savers' Exchange (SSE)
3076 N. Winn Rd.
Decorah, IA 52101
Grassroots network of gardeners who maintain and distribute over five thousand heirloom and rare varieties of food crops, $1 brochure, $25 membership.

Shepherd's Garden Seeds
7389 Zayante
Felton, CA 95018
Retail catalog $1, and bulk price list.

Southern Exposure Seed Exchange
P.O. Box 158
North Garden, VA 22959
Catalog $3, heirlooms, some organic, and seed-saving supplies.

Taylor's Herb Gardens, Inc.
1535 Lone Oak Rd.
Visa, CA 92083
Large selection of medicinal herb seedlings, ships nationwide.

Territorial Seed Company
P.O. Box 157
Cottage Grove, OR 97424
Specializing in varieties for the Pacific Northwest.

Thompson & Morgan, Inc.
P.O. Box 1308
Jackson, NJ 08527
Hard-to-find flower cultivars.

Vesey's Seeds Ltd.
P.O. Box 9000
Calais, ME 04619
Selections for cold climates.

William Dam Seeds, Ltd.
P.O. Box 8400
Dundas, Ontario, Canada L9H6M1
Catalog $2, interesting selections, especially flowers.

Yearly Moon Calendars

Llewellyn's Organic Gardening Almanac, Gardening by the Moon, edited by Mary Wynne. St. Paul, MN: Llewellyn Publications.
I use this book every day to guide my gardening work. There are interesting and educational articles in the book as well as exact planting times and dates for various kinds of plants for the whole year.

The Lunar Calendar, Dedicated to the Goddess in Her Many Guises, edited by Nancy F. W. Passmore. Boston, MA: Luna Press.
A wonderful monthly moon calendar to hang on your wall. Each month depicts the changing moon's phases and lists astrological information.

We'Moon, edited by Musawa. Estacada, OR: Mother Tongue Ink.
A beautiful, inspiring book filled with many different women's quotes and artwork, monthly astrological and herbal information, and a day-by-day astrological calendar.

Homeopathic Organizations

American Holistic Veterinary Medical Association
2214 Old Emmorton Rd.
Bel Air, MD 21014
(301) 838-7778

International Association for Veterinary Homeopathy
General Secretary and Editorial Office
Dr. J. van der Heul
Bestratt 7
9501 HV Stadskannal, The Netherlands

International Foundation for Homeopathy
1141 NW Market St.
Seattle, WA 98107

National Center for Homeopathy
801 North Fairfax St. Suite 306
Alexandria, VA 22314
(703) 548-7790
Contact the center to find a homeopathic study group in your area.

SUPPLIERS OF HOMEOPATHIC REMEDIES

Boiron-Borneman
Box 54
Norwood, PA 19074
(800) BLU-TUBE

Hahneman Medical Clinic Pharmacy
828 San Pablo Ave.
Albany, CA 94706
(510) 527-3003
  Sells to health care providers.

Standard Homeopathic Company
P.O. Box 61067
Los Angeles, CA 90061
(800) 624-9659

Washington Homeopathic Pharmacy
4914 Del Ray Ave.
Bethesda, MD 20814
(800) 336-1695

Naturopathic Doctors
To find a naturopathic doctor in your area, call the American Association of Naturopathic Physicians at (206) 323-7610.

Notes

INTRODUCTION

1. Dawson, Adele. *Herbs: Partners in Life.* Rochester, VT: Healing Arts Press, 1991, p. xi.

CHAPTER 1

1. Reis, Patricia. *Through the Goddess: A Woman's Way of Healing.* New York, NY: Continuum Publishing, 1991, pp. 14–15.
2. Banton, Michael. *Witchcraft, Confessions, and Accusations.* London, Eng.: Tavistock Publications, 1970, p. 2.
3. Ehrenreich, Barbara, and Deirdre English. *For Her Own Good: 150 Years of the Experts' Advice to Women.* New York, N.Y.: Doubleday, 1979, p. 35.
4. Banton, op. cit.
5. Ibid.
6. Griggs, Barbara. *Green Pharmacy: A History of Herbal Medicine.* New York, NY: Viking Press, 1981, p. 175.
7. Achterberg, Jeanne. *Woman as Healer.* Boston, MA: Shambala, 1990, p. 141.
8. Coulter, Harris L. *Divided Legacy: The Conflict Between Homeopathy and the American Medical Association.* Richmond, CA: North Atlantic Books, 1973, p. 93.
9. Achterberg, op. cit., p. 156.
10. This information came from herbalist David Winston, founder of Herbalist and Alchemist, in a phone conversation with the author in April 1994.
11. Boston Women's Health Book Collective. *The New Our Bodies, Ourselves.* New York, NY: Simon & Schuster, 1992, p. 666.
12. Ibid, p. 669.

CHAPTER 3

1. Duke, James A., and Steven Foster. *Peterson Field Guides: Eastern/Central Medicinal Plants.* Boston, MA: Houghton Mifflin, 1990, p. 194.

2. Foster, Steven. *Herbal Renaissance: Growing, Using and Understanding Herbs in the Modern World.* Salt Lake City, UT: Gibbs Smith, 1984, p. 65.
3. Walker, Barbara G. *The Woman's Dictionary.* San Francisco, CA: Harper and Row, 1988, p. 488.
4. Ibid.
5. Spretnak, Charlene. *Lost Goddesses of Early Greece: A Collection of Pre-Hellenic Myths.* Boston, MA: Beacon Press, 1981, p. 69.
6. Weiss, Rudolf Fritz. *Herbal Medicine.* Beaconsfield, Eng.: Beaconsfield Publishers, 1988, p. 32.

CHAPTER 4

1. Schechter, Steven R. *Fighting Radiation With Food, Herbs, and Vitamins.* Brookline, MA: East West Health Books, 1988, p. 78.
2. Ibid., p. 72.
3. Ibid.
4. This information came from biologist Dr. Ryan Drum in a conversation with the author in Maine in August 1991.
5. Schechter, op. cit., p. 76.
6. Drum, op. cit.
7. Teas, Jane. "The Consumption of Seaweed as a Protective Factor in the Etiology of Breast Cancer." *Medical Hypotheses* 7 (5): 601–613.
8. Schechter, op. cit., p. 175.
9. Ibid., p. 70.

CHAPTER 5

1. Hobbs, Christopher. *Foundations of Health: The Liver and Digestive Herbal.* Capitola, CA: Botanica Press, 1992, p. 229.
2. *Wall Street Journal,* October 30, 1991.

CHAPTER 6

Chapter Opener, p. 95. Clear spring water pours from these vaginally-shaped rocks into a sacred pool which Buddhists visit every 28 days and leave offerings in honor of divine female energy. Drawn from a photograph taken by the author in Nepal.
1. Noble, Vicki. *Shakti Woman.* New York, NY: HarperCollins, 1991, p. 31.
2. Reis, Patricia. *Through the Goddess: A Woman's Way of Healing.* New York, NY: Continuum Publishing, 1991, p. 54.

3. Willis, Janice. *Femine Ground: Essays on Women and Tibet.* Ithaca, NY: Snow Lion Publications, 1987, pp. 57–61.
4. This information came from a class handout compiled by Christine Northrup, M.D.
5. Lark, Susan. *Premenstrual Syndrome Self-Help Book.* Los Angeles, CA: Forman Publishing, 1984, p. 77.
6. Ibid., p. 80.
7. Ibid.
8. Weiss, Rudolf Fritz. *Herbal Medicine.* Beaconsfield, Eng: Beaconsfield Publishers, 1988, p. 318.
9. Ibid., p. 318.
10. Foster, Steven, and Yue Chongxi. *Herbal Emissaries: Bringing Chinese Herbs to the West.* Rochester, VT: Healing Arts Press, 1992, p. 66.
11. Kaminski, Patricia, and Richard Katz. *Flower Essence Repertory.* Nevada City, CA: Flower Essences Services, 1992, p. 187.

Chapter 7

Chapter Opener, p. 137. "Goddess Burl Tree." The rounded and full curves on this tree are similar to the many figurines with egg-shaped buttocks and large breasts and hips which archaeologist Marija Gimbutas unearthed and wrote about in *The Language of the Goddess.* Drawn from a photograph taken by the author in Maine.

Chapter 8

1. Brigham and Women's Hospital Study. *Cancer.* July 15, 1982. See also D. L. Longo and R. C. Young, "Cosmetic Talc and Ovarian Cancer," *Lancet,* volume 2 (August 1979).
2. This information came from Peaches Bass, a women's health researcher, in a conversation with the author in May 1994.
3. Lichtman, Bonnie, and Susan Papera. *Gynecology: Well-Woman Care.* Norwalk, CT: Appleton and Longe, 1990, p. 187.
4. Boston Women's Health Book Collective. *The New Our Bodies, Ourselves.* New York, NY: Simon & Schuster, 1984, p. 270.
5. Ibid., revised ed., 1992, p. 607.
6. Ibid., p. 318.
7. Ibid., p. 573.
8. Ibid.
9. Johnson, Susan R., Elaine M. Smith, and Susan M. Guenther. "Comparison of Gynecological Health Care Problems Between

Lesbians and Bisexual Women." *The Journal of Reproductive Medicine*, vol. 32, number 11, November 1987.

CHAPTER 9

1. *Women's Health: Readings on Social, Economic & Political Issues.*
2. Boston Women's Health Book Collective. *The New Our Bodies, Ourselves.* New York, NY: Simon & Schuster, 1992, p. 597.
3. Ibid., 1984 ed., p. 511.
4. Ibid., p. 513.
5. Ibid., 1992 ed., p. 593.
6. O'Doneell, Mary, Kater Pollock, Val Leoffler, and Siesel Saunders. *Lesbian Health Matters.* Santa Cruz, CA: Santa Cruz Women's Health Center, 1979, p. 100.

CHAPTER 10

Chapter Opener, p. 225. A Tamang woman from Nepal. This ethnic group lives in the high hills surrounding the Kathmandu valley.
1. Doress, Paula Brown; Diana Laskin Siegal; and the Midlife and Older Women Book Project. *Ourselves, Growing Older.* New York, NY: Simon & Schuster, 1987, p. xiv.
2. This information came from Dr. Mary Lynn Garner during a class on menopause attended by the author in April 1994.
3. This information came from Dr. Christine Northrup in a conversation with the author in October 1990.
4. Ibid.
5. MacDonald, Barbara, and Cynthia Rich. *Look Me in the Eye.* San Francisco, CA: Spinsters/Aunt Lute Book Company, 1983; reprinted in *Women's Health: Readings on Social, Economic and Political Issues*, p. 104.
6. Nearing, Helen. *Loving and Leaving the Good Life.* Post Mills, VT: Chelsea Green Publishing, 1992, p. 194.

CHAPTER 11

1. Hobbs, Christopher. "A New Strategy for Rebuilding Immunity." *Vegetarian Times*, November 1989, pp. 72–75.
2. Ibid.

GLOSSARY

Common English Names	Latin Names
Alfalfa	*Medicago sativa*
Angelica	*Angelica archangelica*
Anise hyssop	*Agastache foeniculum*
Arnica	*Arnica montana*
Astragalus	*Astragalus membranaceus*
Basil, Sacred	*Ocimum sanctum*
Balm, Bee	*Monarda sp.*
Balm, Lemon	*Melissa officinalis*
Bearberry	*Arctostaphylos uva-ursi*
Bethroot	*Trillium erectum*
Blackberry	*Rubus occidentalis*
Black cohosh	*Cimicifuga racemosa*
Black walnut	*Juglans nigra*
Black Haw	*Viburnum prunifolium*
Bladderwrack	*Fucus vesiculosus*
Blessed thistle	*Cnicus benedictus*
Blue cohosh	*Caulophyllum thalictroides*
Boneset	*Eupatorium perfoliatum*
Borage	*Borago officinalis*
Buckwheat	*Fagopyrum esculentum*
Burdock	*Arctium lappa*
Calamus	*Acorus americanus*
Calendula	*Calendula officinalis*
Catnip	*Nepeta cataria*
Chamomile	*Matricaria recutita*
Chasteberry	*Vitex agnus-castus*
Chickweed	*Stellaria media*
Cleavers	*Galium aparine*
Cinnamon	*Cinnamomum sp.*

Codonopsis	*Codonopsis sp.*
Comfrey	*Symphytum officinale*
Corn silk	*Zea mays*
Crampbark	*Viburnum opulus*
Daisy, English	*Bellis perennis*
Dandelion	*Taraxacum officinale*
Dong Quai	*Angelica sinensis*
Dulse	*Palmaria palmata*
Echinacea	*Echinacea purpurea*
Eyebright	*Euphrasia sp.*
False unicorn	*Chamaelirium luteum*
Fennel	*Foeniculum officinalis*
Fenugreek	*Trigonella foenum-grecum*
Feverfew	*Tanacetum parthenium*
Garlic	*Allium sativum*
Gentian	*Gentiana sp.*
Ginger	*Zingiber officinalis*
Ginkgo	*Ginkgo biloba*
Ginseng	*Panax quinquefolius*
Goldenseal	*Hydrastis canadensis*
Hawthorn	*Crataegus sp.*
Heartsease pansy	*Viola tricolor*
Hops	*Humulus lupulus*
Horehound	*Marrubium vulgare*
Horsetail	*Equisetum arvense*
Hyssop	*Hyssopus officinalis*
Kelp	*Laminaria longicruris*
Lady's mantle	*Alchemilla vulgaris*
Lavender	*Lavandula officinalis*
Lemon balm	*Melissa officinalis*
Lemon verbena	*Aloysia triphylla*
Linden	*Tilia sp.*
Licorice	*Glycyrrhiza glabra*
Lomatium	*Lomatium dissectum*
Meadowsweet	*Spirea latifolia*
Milk thistle	*Silybum marianum*
Motherwort	*Leonurus cardiaca*
Mullein	*Verbascum thapsus*
Nettle	*Urtica dioica*

Oats	*Avena sp.*
Ocotillo	*Fouquieria splendens*
Partridge berry	*Mitchella repens*
Parsley	*Petroselinum sativum*
Pasque flower (Pulsatilla)	*Anemone pulsatilla*
Passion flower	*Passiflora incarnata*
Peach leaves	*Amygdalus persica*
Peppermint	*Mentha piperita*
Plantain	*Plantago major*
Pipsissewa	*Chimaphila umbellata*
Poke	*Phytolacca decandra*
Polygala	*Polygala tenuifolia*
Prickly ash	*Zanthoxylum clava-herculis*
Raspberry	*Rubus idaeus*
Red clover	*Trifolium pratense*
Rosemary	*Rosmarinus officinalis*
Rose petals and hips	*Rosa rugosa*
Sarsaparilla	*Smilax sp.*
Saw palmetto	*Sabal serrulata*
Schizandra	*Schizandra chinensis* or *Schizandra splenanthera*
Shepherd's purse	*Capsella bursa-pastoris*
Siberian ginseng	*Eleutherococcus senticosus*
Skullcap	*Scutellaria lateriflora*
Southernwood	*Artemesia abronatum*
Spilanthes	*Spilanthes acmella*
St. Johnswort	*Hypericum perforatum*
Thuja	*Thuja occidentalis*
Thyme	*Thymus sp.*
Ti tree	*Melaleuca alternifolia*
Usnea	*Usnea sp.*
Valerian	*Valeriana officinalis*
Vervain, Blue	*Verbena officinalis*
White ash	*Fraxinus americana*
Wild yam	*Dioscorea quaternata* or *villosa*
Wormwood	*Artemesia absinthum*
Yarrow	*Achillea millefolium*
Yellow birch	*Betula lutea*
Yellow dock	*Rumex crispus*

Index to Herbal Formulas

General Index

Diarrhea, 49, 91, 118, 122
*Difficult Decision: A Compassionate Book
About Abortion, A* (Gardner), 140
Digestion, 74–75
    stimulant, 122
Digestive system, 86–87, 111
    alfalfa, 45
    calendula, 47
    chamomile, 49
    chickweed, 51
    herbal formulas, 88–90, 160, 163
    lemon balm, 55
    stomach cramps, 49
Dioscorea villosa. See Wild yam
Diuretic, 78
Diverticulitis, 121
Dong Quai, 112–13, 127, 130, 133, 139, 141,
    148, 188, 211–12, 216, 234, 244
Dr. Susan Love's Breast Book, 214
Drying herbs, 26–27
Dulse, 66–68, 70, 104
Duodenal ulcers, 47
Dusty miller, 247
Dysentery, 122

Echinacea, 38, 252–53, 255
    bacterial vaginosis, 165–67
    benign breast condition, 217
    cataract surgery, 248
    chlamydia, 184
    CIN, 177
    condyloma, 181
    in eyewash, 52
    herpes, 172
    hysterectomy, 210
    trichomonas, 162–63
    urinary tract infection, 221
    and vaccination, 258
    vaginal suppositories, 167, 179
    yeast infections, 157
Eclectics, 17, 19
Eczema, 47, 52, 57, 61, 76, 82
Elder, 122
Elliot, Doug, 108, 235
Emmenagogues, 130–31
Endometriosis, 109, 114, 194–201
    dietary support, 196
    herbal formulas, 197–200
    supplements, 197
    treatments, 195–96
Environmental illnesses, 259–61
Environmental pollution, 67
Epileptic seizures, 59
Erhart, Linnette, 68
Erhart, Shep, 69

Escharotic treatment, 179–80, 184
Estrogen, 110, 113
Exercise during menopause, 228–29, 243
Eyebright, 52, 247–48
Eyes, 47, 52
    cataract remedies, 247–48

Face steams, 42
False unicorn, 112, 113–14, 121, 127
    chlamydia, 185
    endometriosis, 198
    estrogen replacement therapy, 244
    menopause, 234, 237
    miscarriage, 139, 141
    postpartum, 148
Fennel, 57, 74, 88, 90, 120, 142, 150, 236,
    248
Fennugreek, 236
Fertility, 68, 114, 121
    herbal formula, 138–39
Fever, 55, 61, 122
    Fever/Flu Remedy, 258–59
Feverfew, 114–16, 134
Fibrocystic breast tissue, 68
    herbs for decreasing, 216
Flagyl, 163, 167
Flatulent dyspepsia, 55
Flax-seed oil, 156, 170, 175, 182, 184, 197,
    207, 210, 215, 220, 231, 251
Floradix, 132–33, 142, 197
Flower Essence Repertory, The, 123
Flower essences, 33–36, 205
    Bach Flower Essences, 34
    cauliflower, 145
    choosing, 36
    diluting, 35–36
    hawthorn, 190
    how to make, 34–35
    Rescue Remedy. *See* Rescue Remedy
    yarrow, 123
Flu, 61, 122, 252
    Fever/Flu Remedy, 258–59
Folic acid, 175
Fomentation. *See* compress
*Foundations of Health: The Liver and Digestive
    Herbal* (Hobbs), 74
Fragrine, 62
Fucus, 66
Fungus. *See* Yeast infections

Gallbladder, 47, 78, 81, 121
Gardner, Joy, 140
Gardnerella. *See* Bacterial vaginosis
Garlic, 38, 158, 231
Garner, Mary Lynn, 231